RUN AWAY FROM FAT

The 90-Day Weight-Loss Program

Dave Kuehls

A Perigee Book

A Perigee Book
Published by The Berkley Publishing Group
A member of Penguin Putnam Inc.
375 Hudson Street
New York, New York 10014

Copyright © 1999 by Dave Kuehls
Cover design by Miguel Santana
Interior design by Lisa Stokes
Cover photos © by Ariel Skelley/The Stock Market; © by Paul Steel/The Stock Market; © by David Madison/Tony Stone Images; © by Chad Slattery/Tony Stone Images
Interior illustrations by Pat Dougherty

First edition: April 1999

Published simultaneously in Canada.

The Penguin Putnam Inc. World Wide Web site address is
http://www.penguinputnam.com

Library of Congress Cataloging-in-Publication Data

Kuehls, Dave.
     Run away from fat : the 90-day weight-loss program / Dave Kuehls.
        p.   cm.
     ISBN 0-399-52485-1
     1. Weight loss.   2. Running.   I. Title.
   RM222.2.K83   1999
   613.7'172—dc21   98-50210
                                                                          CIP

Printed in the United States of America

10   9   8   7   6   5   4   3   2   1

INTRODUCTION

I T HAPPENED my second year of graduate school. I got on the scale and—whoo! Where did those seven extra pounds come from?

I was studying quite a bit. Perhaps eating more junk food—and drinking more beers—than I should have. But that wasn't the real reason why, at 24, I had expanded my belt size by an inch and a half.

Let's backtrack. I had always been a runner. I ran in junior high, high school, captained my college cross-country team and during my first year of graduate school I'd found a good training partner and we were running 5–8 miles a day 5 to 6 times a week. But this year my training partner was too busy to run on a regular basis and so I slacked off too. The evenings I used to spend down at the track or on the trail, I found myself hanging out in coffee shops or movie theaters. Soon I was down to running three times a week, then two, then not at all.

I gained weight: A water-balloon-like rim of fat around my belt line, where most men gain weight (women tend to store fat in the back of the legs). I didn't like what I saw and didn't like how I felt (though I wasn't running at all, I had less energy). So I called up my ex–training partner. The conversation went something like this:

> Me: I've put on 7 pounds this semester.
> Eric: I've put on 6.
> Me: How about I meet you at the trail tomorrow about five-thirty? We'll run an easy half hour to start.
> Eric: I'll be there.

By the end of the semester we'd both run away from fat and got back down to our ideal weights. And ever since, when work gets in the way and I slack off and I start to see the weight creep back on, I remind myself to start running more regularly, and the fat melts off like a stick of butter on a hot grill.

That's my testimonial. Throughout this book you'll read eleven other testimonials from people who've lost anywhere from a few pounds to more than 100 pounds through running.

Why running? Because it is the most efficient fat burner on the planet. It burns more fat in less time than walking, cycling, aerobics or any newfangled device that they're trying to sell you with an infomercial. It's also darn easy to do. All you need is a good pair of shoes and the willpower to take that first step. And perhaps a guide to take you through the first months. Presumably that's why you bought this book: Because you want to lose weight, and you want to do it by running. But you need a little help with information and motivation.

The goal of this book is more than just to help you to lose weight by getting you to run for 90 days. The goal is to introduce you to a new lifestyle—the running lifestyle—where you fit in a run several times a week and keep burning fat for the rest of your life. Because you'll find that once you lose the weight you want to, running is the best way to keep it off.

HOW TO USE THIS BOOK

THE 90-DAY Run Away From Fat Program is your guide to losing weight and becoming a runner. If you follow the program, by the end of 90 days you'll be running up to 40 minutes a day. Forty minutes is a good goal because in 40 minutes you can not only burn a lot of fat and calories, but 40 minutes of running also gives your heart and lungs a good workout, making you more fit—and able to run farther in the future, and burn more fat and calories. (At the end of 90 days you'll also know five key Fat-Burning Runs that you can use to maximize weight loss.)

This book is designed to be read one day at a time. Each day will outline your running goal—for example, 10 minutes to start—and cover a topic that is important to burning fat and calories or making you a better runner overall. At the end of each day you will find a log where you can record your run for that day and any other comments you want to make.

As the days increase, so will your running time. You might notice a staggered increase—that is, you don't go directly from running 10 minutes to 20 minutes to 30 minutes to 40 minutes. You'll run 20 minutes one day and then the next day you might run only 10 minutes. This is for a good reason. Each time you run farther you are stressing the body so that it will need a day or two to re-cover, to grow stronger. If you don't do this and jump from 10 minutes to 20 to 30 to 40, you're setting yourself up to get injured.

Of course, there will be a few of you who can already do this program. For you, you can try doubling the minutes each day. For some others there may be days you're more tired than usual (there will be one day of rest each week) and you can't quite meet the 20 minutes of running outlined as the goal for that day. This is okay. The book is a rough guideline for you. It is not etched in stone. The important thing is to stay consistent, to keep running 6 days a week. And if you can only run 15 minutes on a day when 20 is scheduled, that is fine. But try to stay as close to the schedule as possible. (If you can't come close, try cutting the running time in half for each day. Therefore, you'll be running 20 minutes at the end of 90 days, instead of 40 minutes.)

The important thing is to get out there and *Run Away from Fat.*

10 MINUTES

Today's Run

For your first run find a flat trail or deserted road and run "out" for five minutes, then "back" for five minutes. Don't worry about going fast. Just keep moving for 10 minutes.

Testimonial

MEET CARRIE. She's a 24-year-old medical student. She's bright, attractive and . . . slim. To look at her, you wouldn't have guessed her secret.

"I weighed 80 pounds more than this a year ago," she says.

It all started one winter day when Carrie decided to make a change. "I had tried diets but they didn't get the job done," she says. "I exercised some, but it wasn't on a regular basis. I told myself this time I was going to get on a running program and stick to it."

It was hard at first. "But I made runs my first priority each day," she recalls. "It was what came before everything else."

Carrie ran 5 or 6 days a week and soon she was up to her goal time—40 minutes of running a day. "If it was nice I went outside," she says. "If it was bad weather or I got home too late to run outside I got on a treadmill and did it. I told myself I just wanted to get in 40 minutes each day."

Sure, there were times when she couldn't run very fast and didn't. "I just told myself to keep moving for 40 minutes," she recalls. "That was the goal."

She also watched what she ate, and soon the fat was melting away. "It didn't start right away, but when it did the weight came off real fast," she says.

Five pounds!

Ten pounds!

Twenty pounds!

Forty pounds!

Eighty pounds!

Eighty pounds later, Carrie looks back at the year that was, then looks down at her new body.

"Running was the key, but the other key was that I was ready to do it," she says. "I was ready to commit."

Are you ready to make the commitment?

Day One Log

Time: _____

Place: _____

Comments: _____

_____

_____

10 MINUTES

Today's Run

Out for five minutes and back for five minutes.

Running Technique

Running is one of the easiest exercises to learn and master. You just need to get out the door and do what you did when you were a kid—run.

Here are some tips on running form:

1. Your head: Should be straight up and down or slightly leaning forward. If your head arches back, you'll throw the rest of your body off balance and will be working against yourself, as if you're continuously running uphill. If your head is too far forward you will be shortening your stride—taking baby steps—because your body is hunched forward and is too compact.

2. Your mouth: Breathe in and out through a comfortably open mouth. Some people like to breathe in through the nose, then out through the mouth.

3. The lower lip: Loose. If you have a loose lower lip, that means you're not clenching your teeth. And the rest of your body stays loose, too.

dave kuehls

4 Shoulders: Loose rather than tight. Upright or with a slight forward lean. Be sure not to hunch your shoulders.

5 Arms: Bent perpendicular at the elbow. Swing back and forth between the waist and the bottom of your rib cage. Give yourself a couple of inches' berth on each side so you're not punching yourself in the kidneys with each swing.

6 Hands: Half-fists. Do not clench. Keep them between waist level and rib-cage level. Pump them lower and harder when going uphill.

7 Thumbs: Keep loose and outside the fist.

8 Back: Upright or slight forward lean.

9 Chest: Upright.

10 Lungs: Learn to belly breathe. That is, take deep breaths and push down with your diaphragm, expanding the stomach, not the chest. Breathing this way ensures that you are inflating the lungs with each breath.

11 Hips: Forward and under you.

12 Butt: Forward and under.

13 Knees: Gentle lift but not pronounced. You should not feel your knee lift in the thigh muscles, unless you are sprinting or running uphill.

14 Leg swing: Reach out just ahead of you to land, and swing your leg back behind you—your foot going halfway up toward your butt. Don't reach out too far. That means you are over-

striding (slowing yourself down by taking steps that are too big).

15 Foot placement: Land on your heel, roll to the front of your foot, and push off with the ball of your foot, not your toes.

These are the basic rules for running. But one rule supersedes all others:

Do what feels natural.

The perfect technique for you might not be the one you see on great runners or even friends who are running with you. Use the technique that feels best for you. If it's comfortable and feels right, you'll keep running.

Day Two Log

Time: _____

Place: _____

Comments: _____

_____

_____

10 MINUTES

Today's Run

Out for five minutes and back for five minutes.

Why Diets Alone Don't Work

We all know someone who went on a diet—maybe you've been on a diet, too—and lost some weight, maybe a lot of weight, only to gain it right back in a matter of weeks or months.

DRASTICALLY CUTTING back on the amount of calories you consume doesn't work for two major reasons:

1 Dieting slows the metabolism. Your metabolism is the fire in your belly that burns calories. By starving yourself by dieting, you're taking fuel away from the fire, so eventually it dies down. When you decide to eat again, you'll pack it on faster than you can say thunder thighs or beer belly, because your metabolism has been effectively turned off, like the burner on a stove.

2 Dieting is not a long-range plan. Sooner or later you're going to want to eat.

By dieting or reducing calories, you'll starve yourself at breakfast, starve yourself at lunch, starve yourself at dinner and go to bed so hungry you dream of deep-dish pizzas covered in ice cream. For a while dieting works. You will lose weight but it won't stay off.

Deprivation diets last for finite periods of time—the five-day diet-diet, the two-week diet, etc. And that's for a good reason. No one has the willpower to deny themselves food for much longer. So, in a way, those diets are really a trick, a witch's spell to be 16 again, but two weeks later you're back to your old self.

The "rebound effect" of dieting—when you gain back the pounds you've lost (often more)—won't happen if you combine a sensible eating program with the running program outlined in this book. That's because running with sensible eating is not a quick fix that will spring more than a few leaks sooner or later.

Run Away from Fat presents a long-term plan for losing weight and keeping it off for the rest of your life.

Though the book's time frame is 90 days, it does not end at 90 days (you won't be clothes-hanger thin or so weak from lack of food that you're ready to gorge yourself if someone will just help you to the buffet line). Instead, it's only a beginning.

Think of it as the first 90 days of the rest of your life.

It's the start of a lifetime of maintaining a healthy, trim body through running, the best such exercise to do so.

Day Three Log

Time: _____

Place: _____

Comments: _____

_____

_____

10 MINUTES

Today's Run

Out for five minutes and back for five minutes.

Shoes

■ ■ ■ ■ ■ ■ ■ ■ ■ ■ ■

WHEN YOU run, your feet hit the ground with a force up to four times your body weight. That's quite a shock and in order to prevent aches, pains and injuries, you need a good pair of running shoes.

What makes a good pair of running shoes?

The most important criteria is that they are comfortable to you. Try on a pair in the shoe store. Walk or jog in them through the aisles. Is there enough room for your toes? Does the back of the shoe rub against your heel? How does the top of your foot feel against the laces?

These are the major questions that need answering before you take that pair home with you.

Another consideration is price. Some shoes cost more than $100 a pair. While you don't need to spend that much on a pair of running shoes, you should know that a decent pair of running shoes is going to cost at least $50 (look for the known brands like

New Balance, Nike, Reebok, Adidas). Pay any less and the shoes you'll be getting won't last through the 90-day schedule. They're more for the weekend runner or people who run once or twice a week. Not people who run five or six times a week like you.

If you are a bulky runner, consider buying special running shoes that are made for "motion control." What that means is that these shoes are built to keep your feet and ankles stable, so when you run you are going forward, not wavering to the sides.

You also might consider buying a second pair of shoes sometime after the first week (when you're sure you've found the right pair). The second pair will be worn every other day and will make both pairs last longer, increasing the shock-absorbing potential of both. (There are few things worse than plodding around on a worn-out pair of shoes. You might as well be running on cardboard.)

Day Four Log

Time: _____

Place: _____

Comments: _____

_____

_____

10 MINUTES

Today's Run

Out for five minutes and back for five minutes.

Clothing

■ ■ ■ ■ ■ ■ ■ ■ ■ ■ ■ ■ ■ ■ ■

BESIDES A good pair of running shoes, there are some other essential items of clothing you'll need:

1. Shorts. You'll need comfortable shorts or sweatpants. They should be loose and preferably not cotton—cotton gets soggy when you sweat. Standard running shorts are made by all the major running shoe companies. But you can also wear soccer shorts (more room) or walking shorts (as long as they don't bind). Wear whatever feels comfortable.

   The best part about wearing running shorts or soccer shorts is that you can wash them every day. Just take them into the shower with you and then rinse them off and hang them up to dry. By the time tomorrow's run is scheduled, they'll be ready to wear.

2. Socks. Socks should be white (colors bleed when you sweat) and preferably of ankle length. Avoid tube socks that stretch up over the calf. They'll only droop when the elastic loses its grip. Buy 3–4 pairs and always run in a clean pair. Running in dirty socks is an invitation to athlete's foot. Look for "running socks" at the shoe store.

3 Top. A T-shirt can suffice on more temperate days; just make sure it's loose. Some heavier runners feel comfortable wearing two T-shirts at one time, one larger one over another shirt. Again, just wear what feels comfortable to you (just don't dress up so much that you are overheated). Also, don't wear a T-shirt with a lot of stiff lettering on the front. Sometimes that can cause a chafing problem on your chest and sides.

4 Watch. You'll need a watch for this program. It doesn't have to be a fancy sports watch, but you need to be able to tell time by the minutes very easily (you'll be looking on the run). If you buy a sports watch, try the stopwatch function first. It should be easy to press the buttons to stop and start, and the seconds and minutes on the timer should be large.

5 Underwear. Most running shorts come with briefs built in. If you run in soccer shorts or walking shorts, you might consider wearing a pair of running shorts underneath. They're better than cotton briefs because they're built to absorb moisture and won't bind. For women, a "jog bra" is recommended to wear under your T-shirt. It's more sturdy than the normal bra, giving you more support.

6 Optional items. Hats and sunglasses are optional. If you feel comfortable wearing them, use them. A "fanny pack" to carry water might come in handy on some of your runs over 30 minutes. But on short runs leave it behind. It's only excess weight that will hinder your progress.

Day Five Log

Time: _____

Place: _____

Comments: _____

_____

_____

10 MINUTES

Today's Run

Out for five minutes and back for five minutes.

Why Running Is the Best Exercise to Lose Weight

A NY EXERCISE is better than no exercise at all. But among exercises there is a hierarchy, a list of those exercises that burn more calories and fat per minute than others.

Running is at the top.

For example, a 160-pound man running at a good clip will burn 547 calories in a half hour. Compare that to other exercises:

Stairclimber: 432 calories per half hour.
Cycling: 340 calories per half hour.
Swimming: 336 calories per half hour.
Aerobics: 312 calories per half hour.
Walking: 216 calories per half hour.

Running burns two and a half times more calories in a half an hour than walking does. This makes it the perfect workout for those who are pressed for time. In fact, the faster you run, the more calories you'll burn. (But more on that later.)

For now, we're going to start slow and easy. A nice jog, which is a pace slow enough that your breathing is not taxed. Or a pace that lets you talk freely. (At this pace you'll burn roughly 100 calories every 8–10 minutes. You need to burn off 3,500 calories to lose a pound of fat. And you do this by gradually increasing your run so that you burn more and more each day.)

If you can't jog the full 10 minutes, walk for one minute, then jog for one minute, then walk for one minute until you have completed the 10 minutes.

In addition to a high rate of calorie and fat burning, running is simple. Only walking rivals it in simplicity, and walking, as pointed out, pales in the fat-burning category.

To run, you don't need to wait in line for a lane at the pool, go when an aerobics class is scheduled, or when the stairclimber is open or only when it isn't raining (cycling). When you run you are your own boss, and about the only thing that can stop you from completing your run is an earthquake or typhoon.

One final note: It wouldn't be fair if I didn't mention one exercise that burns as many calories per half hour as running.

That exercise is cross-country skiing. And you can probably guess the hurdles involved in structuring a workout program around cross-country skiing. Especially if you live in Florida.

Day Six Log

Time: _____

Place: _____

Comments: _____

_____

_____

10 MINUTES

Today's Run

Out for five minutes and back for five minutes.

Testimonial

MEET TODD. He's a 32-year-old business executive. Five years ago he weighed 24 pounds more than he does now.

"I weighed 172 pounds when I started a diet program," he recalls. "But dieting alone didn't help that much."

A friend was into running and suggested Todd try it, too, so he decided to buy a pair of shoes and drive down to the local running trail.

"I was intimidated at first," he says. "The trail was 5 miles long and I only made about 2 miles of it. But the great thing about running, I learned, was that if you keep at it, you can go farther just about every week."

Todd ran three miles. Then four miles. Then five miles.

"I was jazzed," he recalls. "The weight was coming off, and running was actually fun. I knew it would help me take the weight off. But I never would have guessed it would be fun."

Today, running at the end of a busy workday is one thing Todd looks forward to. "People who don't run have the wrong idea about running," he says. "They think it's stressful. But they are wrong. It's work that is stressful. Getting out for a relaxing run after work is stress relief. If I don't run, I don't feel as good as when I do run.

"And," Todd adds, "I don't keep the weight off either."

Day Seven Log

Time: _____

Place: _____

Comments: _____

_____

_____

OFF

Today's Run

0 minutes.

Rest Is Good

TODAY IS your first day off. Relax. Put your feet up. Just don't celebrate with a deep-dish pizza and fries. (You should feel your body burning fat. You probably haven't lost any weight or not very much yet, but you're like a runner who is just warming up.)

You need days off. And each week of this program you'll get at least one.

Rest, in fact, is vital—if you want to complete the full 90-day program and propel yourself into the running for fitness life.

If you skip rest days, you're only setting yourself up for an early exit, say, by day 20, because you'll be too tired and sore to go on. And you'll be sick of this running stuff.

Rest days keep your legs and spirit fresh. They recharge both your physical and mental batteries. And they send you on your way to making running an integral part of your fitness life well after the 90 days are up. Rest is, in fact, more important than the hardest runs you'll be doing because during rest the body takes the stress of those workouts and makes your body stronger, so it can handle them again.

It's a principle great athletes in all sports use: Stress and then rest . . . and the body grows stronger.

And it becomes a better fat-burning machine.

Day Eight Log

Time: _____

Place: _____

Comments: _____

_____

_____

15 MINUTES

Today's Run

7 1/2 minutes out, 7 1/2 minutes back.

Increasing Time: 10–20 Minutes

INCREASING THE time you run will be a big step for you, so we are going to take it in two little steps.

By now, you should be feeling comfortable running for 10 minutes at a time. You've worked up from a slow jog to maybe a bit faster pace. Or you are running the entire distance now instead of walk/running.

Now we are going to push forward and go after a common goal for many runners—that is, to run for 20 minutes.

Twenty minutes is a golden number in running because it is the point where your body starts making changes in its energy system. The body actually starts to maximize its ability to burn fat, making fat more likely to come off on a 20-minute run than a 10-minute run.

(Eventually 20 minutes will become a minimal run for you when you've become an accomplished runner and just want to get out for an easy run one day and burn some fat. Twenty minutes is also an amount of time to be proud of—20 minutes is a long time to be doing anything.)

The key to getting to the point where you are running 20 minutes is to think of it in two segments. First run for 15 minutes, then after you are comfortable running for that time, move up to 20 minutes.

You do this by first by adding 2½ minutes onto the "out" portion of your 10-minute run, and 2½ minutes onto the "back" portion of your run.

By adding those few short minutes, you're up to 15 minutes.

Make sure to pick a flat, easy course with not a lot of traffic when you make your attempt at 15 minutes. You want to stack the deck in your favor. Make sure you are rested for these efforts, and you are not hungry—that you have eaten a high-carbohydrate snack 1 or 2 hours before your run.

And, of course, when you are increasing time, it is good to run with a friend.

A final note: Since you will be going longer today, purposely run a step or two slower for the first five minutes, and then work into your normal "talk test" pace [see Day 10]. By easing into your run today you will be giving yourself a psychological edge.

Essentially you'll be buying time that you can tack on to your run at the end—the extra five minutes.

Day Nine Log

Time: _____

Place: _____

Comments: _____

_____

_____

15 MINUTES

Today's Run

Out 7 1/2 minutes, back 7 1/2 minutes.

Take the Talk Test

■ ■ ■ ■ ■ ■ ■ ■ ■ ■ ■ ■ ■ ■

MOST OF your running should be slow enough that you're not stressing your body so much that it can't recover in time for the next day's run. Unless indicated otherwise, all of your runs should be done at this pace.

Which brings up a common problem for world-class runners as well as beginners like yourself: How do I know I am running slowly enough so that I will recover?

One way is to wear a heart monitor and watch that you don't get your heart rate above 65 percent of its maximum.

A much easier way is to take the "talk test."

The "talk test" has been around for years. Essentially what you want to do when you run is to run slowly enough that you can carry on a conversation, without pausing to catch your breath.

If you can talk, you are running slowly enough.

Of course, this means you should be running with a training partner (save all the gossip for your daily runs). And a two-way conversation will keep the pace at the desired level and will also pass the time more quickly.

But what if you are running by yourself on certain days? Do you babble incoherently to yourself about current events and your workday as you run down the trail and hope that no one looks at you sideways?

No, a good way is to count off five seconds every minute looking at your watch. That is, run for a minute and when you get to 60 seconds, look at your watch and count to 5 seconds. If you can do that feeling very comfortable—not puffing air between seconds—your pace is slow enough.

After those 5 seconds keep running at the same pace and then check your watch again at 2 minutes. And count to five. Repeat every minute.

This will keep you on the right pace.

And not make you look like you're one brick shy of a load.

Of course, as you progress, you will learn "pace." You will be able to feel if you're going too fast or too slow and react accordingly.

Day Ten Log

Time: _____

Place: _____

Comments: _____

_____

_____

15 MINUTES

Today's Run

Out 7 1/2 minutes, back 7 1/2 minutes.

That Chafing Problem

O KAY. SO you really don't want to talk about it. It's embarrassing. But you've probably encountered it by now.

Chafing. That rubbing problem on your inner thighs plagues runners of all abilities (U.S. record holder in the marathon Jerry Lawson, chafes because he's bowlegged), but the problem mainly strikes beginning runners who are battling a weight problem. That's because excess fat tends to collect in the thighs and when you run they rub together wearing off the outer layers of skin until you've got a nice circular red spot on both thighs. And it stings.

Eventually, as you slim down, chafing will dissipate and disappear. But for now here's what you can do about it:

1 Apply Vaseline to handle the friction. Glop it over the tender spots right before you run. If you need more, carry a small tube with you on the run.

2 Wear clothes that protect the inner thighs. Biking shorts without the padding—or Tri-Shorts—are made of spandex and they cover the inner thighs. You can wear those underneath your running shorts.

3 Apply a topical antibiotic (such a Neosporin ointment) to the red area to combat infection after you run.

Day Eleven Log

Time: _____

Place: _____

Comments: _____

_____

_____

15 MINUTES

Today's Run

Out 7 1/2 minutes, back 7 1/2 minutes.

Training Log–Use It

T HIS TRAINING log—your training log—is an invaluable tool in running away from fat.

First of all, it helps you track your progress. Each day there is a time goal (say, 15 minutes) and later, a pace (pickups) or training venue goal (such as hills) that you should try to complete.

Fill in the run you did in the space provided each day. Fill it in even if you did not complete the entire run—or did not run as fast or did not run at all. It is important that you make a habit of filling in your log, just as you're making a habit of running six days a week.

The best time to do this is immediately after you come home from your run. Have this book handy with a pen or pencil next to it. You might want to bring it to the park in your car—or down to the health club. The important thing is, fill in your workout each day.

Second, it's a good motivational tool. If you see two or three blank spots in your log in a row (when you didn't run), you'll be more inclined to get out and run. By the same token, if you've stuck with the log for several weeks (what runners call a streak) you'd be less inclined to let yourself slip (especially if you've got all that proof of the good job you've been doing staring back at you in your own handwriting).

Other things you can fill in on your log: How you felt, the weather, your running partner's name, and where and when you ran. A sample entry follows:

Time: 15 minutes
Place: Park this afternoon with Jan
Comments: Beautiful spring day. Feel lighter on my feet than ever before. Weighed myself. Down another pound!

Day Twelve Log

Time: _____

Place: _____

Comments: _____

_____

_____

day thirteen

15 MINUTES

Today's Run

Out 7 1/2 minutes, back 7 1/2 minutes.

The Two-Minute Rule

A S YOU progress in your running program there will be days when you feel plain great. And the workout for that day—say, a 15-minute run—will pass in no time. At the end of the run you'll still feel fresh and you will want to keep going.

This is where the 2-minute rule comes in.

For the first 45 days of this program, if you want to go further than the run scheduled for that day, limit it to an additional two minutes.

The reasoning for this is to keep you running day after day. The run schedule is structured so that you will progress in short steps. If you were to suddenly double your 15-minute run, you would run the risk of being sore or tired the next 2 days—and not running. And maybe on the third day there's extra duty at work, and before you know it you've taken off 4 days in a row. All because you let your enthusiasm get the best of you.

After 45 days you can use the 5-minute rule: If you feel like running more, limit it to an additional 5 minutes.

This extra 2 or 5 minutes will satisfy your craving for more. But it will keep you on the right schedule and thinking about the big picture: running more over a period of months and years to come.

That is how you will run away from fat.

Day Thirteen Log

Time: _____

Place: _____

Comments: _____

_____

_____

15 MINUTES

Today's Run

7 1/2 minutes out, 7 1/2 minutes back.

Testimonial

M EET ELLIE. She's a bright-eyed, attractive 31-year-old registered nurse, but for more than a decade she has struggled to lose weight.

Two years ago she finally decided to try running because many of her coworkers at the hospital were running too.

"At first I could only run for a few minutes at a time," she recalls. "I didn't think I could keep it up. But I decided to hang in there one week at a time."

She kept at it, gradually working her way up to running three to four times a week, two or three miles at a time.

"Within a month I could feel myself losing weight," she says. "And I wanted to lose more."

So she gradually upped her mileage and also began to monitor her diet. "One of the great things about being on a running program is that you want to start living the healthy lifestyle in all parts of your life," she says.

Out went the fatty foods. In went fruits and vegetables. "I love french fries," she says. "But I made a promise to myself: No fatty foods."

By the end of 90 days she had lost 8 pounds. "And it was

pounds that were going to stay off because I had committed myself to running," she says.

Now, a year later, Ellie is 18 pounds lighter and a regular runner.

"I don't think I could have lost the weight without running," she says. "Running got me where I am today."

Day Fourteen Log

Time: _____

Place: _____

Comments: _____

_____

_____

0 MINUTES

Today's Run

0 minutes.

Days Off

▪ ▪ ▪ ▪ ▪ ▪ ▪ ▪ ▪ ▪ ▪ ▪ ▪ ▪ ▪

IN THIS program you get a day off each week—for good reason.

Running is a stress put on your body, and if you are constantly increasing your time and intensity you increase the stress each day. If you keep doing that you'll end up sick or injured and not able to run 90 days or continue much thereafter.

That will be when your weight loss program grinds to a halt.

So we have days off from running.

Use your days off as a training tool to keep you running. Don't fret that you aren't out on the path today. Just make sure to not overeat and you will be fine (also, make sure you eat).

On your days off you should plan some activity to do during you normal run time. If, for example, you run right after work, agree to meet your coworkers and go to an evening movie or have an early dinner at the salad bar. Or use that time to run much-needed errands. Just don't go home and stew because you'll be tempted to go out and run. Of course, if you're feeling tired you might want to go home and put your feet up and watch TV or take a nap. Do it. You deserve it.

On the other hand, if you're raring with energy, you be the best judge. You could sneak in a short run on your day off.

If you do run, limit yourself to 10 minutes. That will give you enough exercise to feel good about yourself without hampering the next day's run.

That is how you make days off easy and productive.

Day Fifteen Log

Time: _____

Place: _____

Comments: _____

_____

_____

20 MINUTES

Today's Run

Out 10 minutes, back 10 minutes. You're jumping up to 20 minutes. Make sure you start nice and easy.

Don't Sweat It: The Myth of Sweat and Weight Loss

WE'VE ALL seen them. People out running in a full sweat suit on a hot day in an effort to lose weight. Or if they don't have a sweat suit on it's three or four shirts or sweatpants because they want to lose weight in their legs through sweat (you can't spot reduce like this because weight loss is a whole-body phenomenon; your body burns fat from where it wants to, not where you want it to).

There's only one thing wrong with this scenario: You don't lose weight through sweat, you lose weight by burning calories.

Sure, you're a few pounds lighter after running 20 minutes in a sweat suit in 85 degree weather (I would never recommend this and vehemently warn you against it), but almost all of that weight loss is water weight. And as soon as you drink until you're not thirsty again, your weight will be right back where it started from. (That's why you don't lose any real weight in a steam bath. Sure, it feels good, but it just drains water from your body, not fat.)

In fact, overdressing to sweat out the pounds is actually counterproductive to weight loss. It can lead to dehydration, which will sap your energy while you run as well as for future runs. And overall it makes running seem like so much of a chore, causing you to cut runs short, when you should be going farther. Or cut them out totally, because it's too hot, especially with a sweatshirt on.

The only way you really lose weight is by running for a longer period of time, and eventually running faster.

So don't put stock in excess sweat. It's the excess exercise that will make you lose the fat.

Day Sixteen Log

Time: _____

Place: _____

Comments: _____

_____

_____

15 MINUTES

Today's Run

Out 7 1/2 minutes, back 7 1/2 minutes.

Fluids

WATER IS an important training tool when you're running to lose weight. If your body runs low you're in danger of being dehydrated and that will cause fatigue, which will cause you to slow down or stop your run. And you might feel so bad that you miss a day or two of running in the future.

Therefore, you should drink lots of fluids. During the day. Before you run. After your run. During you run if it's longer than 30 minutes.

During the Day: Make sure you drink at least six 8-ounce glasses of water each day. A good plan is two glasses in the morning when you get up and your body is naturally dehydrated. (This also helps keep water in you if you like coffee or tea in the morning because coffee and tea will take water from your body. They make you pee.) Then have two glasses with lunch and two glasses with dinner.

Before you run: 30 minutes before your run drink two 8-ounce glasses of water.

After you run: Drink two 8-ounce glasses for every 15 minutes you ran.

You might want to experiment with energy drinks or fluid re-placement drinks. But those contain sugar and calories and are primarily for runners who are competing in longer races.

If you don't feel you need them, why not stick with plain, calo-rie-free water?

Day Seventeen Log

Time: _____

Place: _____

Comments: _____

_____

_____

15 MINUTES

Today's Run

Out 7 1/2 minutes, back 7 1/2 minutes.

Friends

· · · · · · · · · · · · · · · · ·

YOU'RE MORE than two weeks into your running program, feeling pretty good, confident that you can handle the days ahead of you—and the scale shows that you've been making progress with weight loss too.

Now's the time—if you haven't already—to get a friend to join you.

Preferably it should be another person who is trying to lose weight, so you can share your goals.

Running with a friend does several things:

1 It gives you someone to compare notes with. Not just about your runs, but also about your diet. If you both vow to swear off sweets, for instance, running with a friend lets you make daily checks on each other.

2 It gives you an extra reason to get in that run each day. If you know a friend is waiting for you at the trail, track or health club treadmill, you'll be less inclined to skip that day. Your partner is counting on you and soon you will realize that you're not just running for yourself, but for another person too.

③ It makes it fun. Most of the runs in this book are such that you can talk on the way. Let running be your social time. Catch up on things while you're running off the fat.

④ Running with someone can help you get through the tough workouts. Maybe you just don't want to go that extra five minutes—today's run is 15 minutes—and you feel like walking instead. With a running friend by your side to motivate you, you're less likely to stop and walk or stop and sit down. Likewise, when they're ready to stop, you can offer words of encouragement.

⑤ Having a partner can get you through the 90 days. Three months is a long time. And the main reason most people fall off an exercise program like this one is that they lose motivation along the way. It becomes too much of a grind. While these workouts are designed to help ward off the grind, having a friend with you on most days can also help you through it.

Tip: Don't run with your friend every day. But agree to meet three or four times a week. That way you have a few days each week to run on your own, and you'll look forward to running with a friend and telling him or her about your good run the day before.

Day Eighteen Log

Time: _____

Place: _____

Comments: _____

_____

_____

20 MINUTES

Today's Run

Out 10 minutes, back 10 minutes.

What to Eat

■ ■ ■ ■ ■ ■ ■ ■ ■ ■ ■ ■ ■ ■ ■

EVEN IF you are trying to lose weight you need to eat. And you need to know what's best to eat during the 90-Day Run Away From Fat Program.

If you go on a strict diet—one that severely limits your intake of food—and then you try to exercise each day, you're setting yourself up for a very short running program. Perhaps just a couple of days.

That's because you need food—fuel—to help you run way from fat.

The Run Away From Fat Nutritional Program is 4-fold:

1 To supply your body with its running fuel.

2 To eat healthy.

3 To eat regularly.

4 To not overeat.

① Carbohydrates and Fuel: First of all the fuel that you burn for the most part when you run is carbohydrates—breads, cereals, pastas, fruits, vegetables, beans. This is what powers your leg muscles, and the lack of carbohydrate—which should make up approximately 70 percent of your total caloric intake—is what will lead to fatigue on individual runs and days afterward. I repeat: Do not starve yourself and attempt to keep up this running program. You will not last more than a day or two.

(I know what you're thinking: If I'm stuffing myself with carbohydrates and only burning carbohydrates, how do I get rid of the fat on my thighs? First of all you're not going to stuff yourself. Second, while carbohydrate is the main fuel source when you run, you do burn fat also. And, remember, when you run you burn a higher total of calories. This coupled with a smart eating program causes you to lose weight at the end of the day, by making your body turn to its stored fat cells for fuel.)

② Protein and fat round out a healthy diet: By eating a high-carbohydrate meal—say, a plate of pasta with red sauce—you're already eating relatively healthy. But do not try to exist on carbos alone. Your body needs protein (about 25 percent of your diet) and fat (about 5 percent) to help you through each running day. Protein helps in rebuilding leg muscles after a run. And fat is an ally against overeating the bad stuff (if you have a little bit of fat—for instance a piece of low-fat cheese on a turkey sandwich for lunch—you don't crave a lot of it).

We'll cover the third and fourth points on Day 20.

Day Nineteen Log

Time: _____

Place: _____

Comments: _____

_____

_____

15 MINUTES

Today's Run

Out 7 1/2 minutes, back 7 1/2 minutes.

How to Eat

■ ■ ■ ■ ■ ■ ■ ■ ■ ■ ■ ■ ■ ■

S O NOW you're eating carbohydrates as part of a healthy diet. What other things do you need to do?

3 Eat often. By this we do not mean going to the weight lifters' extreme of eating every 90 minutes. The standard three meals a day plus snacks will suffice. Remember this: It hurts you more than helps you when you skip meals. Skipping meals drives up hunger and lowers your metabolism—the fire in your belly that burns fat. And what happens if you skip breakfast is that by the time you get to lunch, you're so hungry you can eat a house and you make bad decisions about what to eat. You pass up the chicken salad and dive right into the double-cheese pepperoni pizza. And all that fat sits in your belly like Buddha.

Also, when you skip meals your blood sugar levels plummet, and you'll feel weak and light-headed when it comes time to run, and you might skip your run too.

4 Breakfast, lunch and dinner should be satiating but not satisfying. By that I mean they should give you energy until your snacks—midmorning, afternoon and an optional evening snack—but not cause you to lean back and pat your belly.

Small meals eaten in tandem with regular healthy snacks (see day 25) keep your metabolism running smoothly and hunger at an even keel.

Remember: You are not on a diet. The idea is not to cut way back on your food or starve yourself silly by just eating soup for a week.

You will not be able to run if you do so. Your goal is to change the way you live, that is, to eat healthy and also burn fat through running.

Day Twenty Log

Time: _____

Place: _____

Comments: _____

_____

_____

20 MINUTES

Today's Run

Out 10 minutes, back 10 minutes.

Testimonial

■   ■   ■   ■   ■   ■   ■   ■   ■   ■   ■   ■   ■   ■

MEET SIMONE. She's a 25-year-old bartender and part-time model.

But five years ago, after her freshman year in college, any sort of modeling career was looking as if it was out of the picture.

"I was your typical college freshman," she says. "I went out a lot and didn't exercise at all. By the end of the year I looked down and I was 15 pounds heavier. I thought to myself: Where did that come from?"

Simone had jogged a bit in high school and that, she soon realized, was what had helped her control her weight.

"I decided to get back into running," she says. "And I'm the kind of person that once I start running, I burn weight fast."

Within three months she had lost the 15 pounds she had gained.

And she learned a lesson. "I now run 4–5 days a week religiously," she says. "I go about 20–25 minutes at a time. It's not that much running but I find that a little running is the best thing to keep the weight off. Cycling, for example, burns some calories too. But it tends to make my legs bigger. Running does not do that.

"And if I want to do any modeling—or just look good at the

beach—I don't want big muscular legs or legs with fat attached to the back. So I run."

Day Twenty-one Log

Time: _____

Place: _____

Comments: _____

_____

_____

0 MINUTES

Today's Run

0 minutes.

Breakfast

A GOOD breakfast will help fuel you through the rest of the day, even a day when you don't run. Breakfast is, as the adage goes, the most important meal of the day. So forget the doughnut and coffee on the way to work. If you don't have time for a healthy breakfast, make time.

Breakfast is also the meal when you should try for a little bit of fat. It will help curb fat cravings later on in the day, and it will also help keep hunger on an even keel. An example of a little fat is a dab of peanut butter on toast. Or a piece of low-fat cheese on a bagel sandwich.

Protein is also something important to have for breakfast. If it is not a part of your regular breakfast, change that habit. Try some skim milk or turkey slices or peanut butter or egg whites. Just don't go with the fried eggs and bacon.

Carbohydrate is also needed at breakfast. Toast, bagels, cereals, fruits. They will give you energy for the rest of the morning.

Finally, don't forget fluids. This is especially important if you're in the coffee habit. A good rule of thumb is to drink two glasses of water when you wake and one glass for every cup of coffee in the morning. The same goes for tea. That's because both are diuretics (they suck water from your body). That's water you will need as sweat on your daily runs.

Sample Breakfasts

Cereal with skim milk
Banana
Orange juice

Toast and a dab of peanut butter
Melon
Coffee
Orange juice and water

Pancakes with a dab of butter and strawberries
Juice

Day Twenty-two Log

Time: _____

Place: _____

Comments: _____

_____

_____

20 MINUTES

Today's Run

Out 10 minutes, back 10 minutes.

Lunch

- - - - - - - - - - - - - - - -

LUNCH PLAYS a crucial role in your running program—getting you ready for your afternoon run.

If you eat too much at lunch you'll feel groggy all afternoon, more ready to take a nap than to go for a 20-minute run. Eat too little and you'll be light-headed and weak and ready to eat rather than run.

The trick is to eat a smart lunch, fueling yourself but not fooling yourself into thinking you need a bag of potato chips or a 16-ounce super slug of soda. Remember: You will get a healthy afternoon snack before your run.

Smart lunchtime eating means protein. That's brain food for your afternoon, giving you energy and enthusiasm.

Carbohydrates are important too, but too many can leave you satiated and groggy. You might think a plate of pasta would be ideal for lunch—it will fuel you through your afternoon run. But more likely than not it will have you looking for a place to nap (carbohydrates can cause drowsiness).

So save the pasta for dinner. Carbohydrates at lunch should be the complex kind—beans, whole grain breads. This increasingly popular carbohydrate burns much slower than the simple sugars in pasta and will give you even energy levels all afternoon.

Also at lunch remember to take in plenty of fluids with your meal (your body uses water to digest food). Watch the coffee and soda intake. Many soft drinks are full of caffeine—robbing you of fluid. Plus, they're almost pure sugar, which will cause a blood sugar drop early in the afternoon and lower energy levels. And all that extra sugar is empty calories that are easily converted to fat.

Sample lunches

Tuna fish sandwich sans mayonnaise on whole grain bread
Water

White chili without the cheese
Carrot sticks
Juice

Bean soup and crackers
Apple
Diet soda

Chicken salad with low-fat dressing
Water

Day Twenty-three Log

Time: _____

Place: _____

Comments: _____

_____

_____

15 MINUTES

Today's Run

Out 7 1/2 minutes, back 7 1/2 minutes.

Dinner

■ ■ ■ ■ ■ ■ ■ ■ ■ ■ ■ ■ ■

DINNER, YOUR post-workout meal, is the time to refuel on carbohydrates—again, without stuffing yourself. You might, happily, find that your "dinnertime" appetite has diminished a bit at this point in your running program. This is one of the wonderful anomalies of running: A running person not only burns more than a sedentary person; he or she often eats less food too.

Dinner should be eaten within an hour after your run, or at least no more than 90 minutes later.

This timing has three very good reasons:

1 The closer to your workout you eat, the higher your metabolism is and the more you will burn.

2 Your appetite will be less if you eat immediately following your run.

3 Pushing dinner off until later in the evening drives up hunger and slows your metabolism. The result: You crave fatty foods, like pizza. And you will stuff yourself on them.

Keep dinner simple. Have the pasta and sauce ready on the counter when you get home. Or stop off on the way home from the gym for takeout Chinese (just watch the fried rice and the egg rolls; if you are feeling particularly hungry, order extra rice).

Sample dinners

Pasta and meat sauce
Salad
Skim milk

Chicken and broccoli over rice
Skim milk

Tuna casserole
Salad
Bread, no butter
Juice

Day Twenty-four Log

Time: _____

Place: _____

Comments: _____

_____

_____

20 MINUTES

Today's Run

Out 10 minutes, back 10 minutes.

Snacks

YOUR DAILY snacks—small, carbohydrate-rich—are as important as your three meals in your Run Away From Fat Program. If you follow a regular schedule—breakfast at 8; lunch at 12:30 and dinner at 7:30—you're going to need something in between meals at 10:30 and 3 o'clock.

That's where a healthy snack comes in. Not doughnuts or strudel in the morning. And not a bag of chips or nachos and cheese in the afternoon.

A healthy snack—a banana, a cup of low-fat yogurt—is good for two reasons: In the morning it keeps you from overeating at lunch. If you skip your snack you'll drive up hunger and have a bad lunch. And in the afternoon your snack helps keep blood sugar levels high so you have energy to burn on your run.

An optional third snack—later at night but not right before bed (it will disrupt sleep) can be eaten . . . if you're hungry. Don't eat just for something to do or out of habit.

Make that snack small and carbohydrate rich. A bowl of cereal with skim milk is a good choice.

The key to snacking is to find the carbohydrate-rich and low-fat snacks that you like: fruit in the morning, pretzels in the afternoon, cornflakes at night. Knowing that you're going to snack

dave kuehls

on these later helps you keep from overeating at mealtimes and eating healthy then too. Instead of having grilled cheese at lunch you say to yourself: No. I'll have the bean soup, and if I'm still hungry I know I'm going to have a bag of pretzels from the vending machine in the afternoon.

A word about your afternoon snack. Many new runners try to phase this one out, thinking that they will burn more fat if they skip this snack and run after work. But in reality all they are doing is setting themselves up to run slower or shorter because they are weak and light-headed because of lack of food.

Suggested snacks

One apple
One banana
Half cup of low-fat yogurt
Half a bagel
4 ounces of pretzels
A small bowl of cereal and skim milk

Day Twenty-five Log

Time: _____

Place: _____

Comments: _____

_____

_____

20 MINUTES

Today's Run

Out 10 minutes, back 10 minutes.

Foods to Avoid

W E ALL have our dietary Achilles heels, foods that are our downfall. For some, it's sweets, for others, fatty snack foods. What follows is a list of the most common trouble foods. Keep running and cut them out of your diet and you'll RUN AWAY FROM FAT.

Pizza

For a long time runners have rewarded themselves with this food. The crust, yes, has carbohydrates, which you need—but that has been canceled out by the fat in the cheese and the sausage and the pepperoni. If pizza is a regular part of your food intake, cut it out (tear out the yellow pages for pizza delivery if it comes to that). If you still can't shake the pizza monkey, try making your own pizza at home. That way you can substitute no-fat cheese for regular cheese and eliminate the high-fat toppings, replacing them with fresh vegetables.

Soft Drinks

Think of soft drinks as empty calories in a can. It's all sugar and many people who drink 2, 3 cans a day are actually adding another meal—a mound of sugar—to their calorie count through soft drinks alone. Not only are the calories bad; the sugar drives up insulin levels and that predisposes your body to store fat. So go with diet drinks or, better yet, plain old water. Diet drinks tend to need a fatty snack food like potato chips or nachos to complete them. Water stands alone.

Alcohol

If you're serious about running away from the fat, one of the best things you can do is cut out alcohol. One glass or wine, one beer, one mixed drink can add up over a period of days. Again, it's worthless calories (alcohol does not fuel runners, contrary to popular myth). And alcohol also interferes with the body's ability to burn fat (it burns alcohol instead). So you could be running more and burning less fat. Substitute light wines and beers. Or simply go with water.

Ice Cream

Ice cream is sugar and fat together, combined in a tasty, easily consumed confection. In short, it's the devil incarnate if you want to run away from fat. Think of sucking down Cokes while you're eating fried cheese sticks. That's ice cream's effect on your thighs and waistline. Substitute ice milk or frozen yogurt.

Sweets

Most of these are taken in such small amounts that we don't think about them too much. But sweets can add up. A cookie, a candy bar, and suddenly we've added another 400 calories to our day—perhaps the 400 calories you'll burn on your run, causing a zero calorie deficit for the day and no weight loss. Get the picture? Substitute sugarless gum or fruit for your sweet tooth.

Day Twenty-six Log

Time: _____

Place: _____

Comments: _____

_____

_____

20 MINUTES

Today's Run

Out 10 minutes, back 10 minutes.

Late-Night Hunger

■ ■ ■ ■ ■ ■ ■ ■ ■ ■ ■ ■ ■ ■ ■ ■ ■ ■

YOU RAN 20 minutes today. Ate a healthy dinner.
It's 10 o'clock. And you wish you had some ice cream.

This is the time many diet experts call crisis time. They tell you to suck it up, drink plenty of water, and go to bed and tough it out until the morning. Some experts recommend you eat nothing after 8 p.m.

This program is not so harsh. You can eat as long as you eat the right things—sorry, no ice cream—and you don't overeat. A good late-night snack is something light, preferably high in carbohydrates (carbohydrates contain tryptophan, an amino acid that helps bring on sleep). Half a bagel is good; so is a bowl of cereal, as long as it's not sugar-coated. Cold pasta left over from dinner can quell hunger pangs. So can a piece of fruit.

Ice cream, chips, cookies are not wise choices at this time, but let's hope that you won't be craving fatty foods because you wisely had a bit of fat to eat during the day. If you do have a weakness for these foods, the secret is not to buy them.

Day Twenty-seven Log

Time: _____

Place: _____

Comments: _____

_____

_____

20 MINUTES

Today's Run

Out 10 minutes, back 10 minutes.

Testimonial

▪ ▪ ▪ ▪ ▪ ▪ ▪ ▪ ▪ ▪ ▪ ▪ ▪ ▪ ▪

Meet Dan. A few years ago this father of two had a hard time walking around the block without stopping to catch his breath.

He decided to run. At first he ran just three times a week, then four, then five. And then the weight started coming off. In four months he had lost 40 pounds. Over the next year he lost 40 more.

Now, 80 pounds later, Dan looks back on how he used to be. "Sure, running got me to lose weight," he says. "But I found that the more I ran, the more I liked it. Running became an important part of my life."

And he got very good at it. Dan started winning road races in his area and eventually moved up to the marathon, where he ran a 3:01 and qualified to run the Boston Marathon.

That's 26.2 miles of running. A great achievement considering where Dan was just a few years before.

"Running has made a dramatic change in my life," says Dan. "Not only have I lost weight, but running has given me a confidence about life that I didn't have before."

Day Twenty-eight Log

Time: _____

Place: _____

Comments: _____

_____

_____

0 MINUTES

Today's Run

0 minutes.

Substitute and Save

IF **YOU** are running almost every day you need to eat healthy and often to keep your energy level up—even on rest days like this one. So where do you eliminate the calories?

The answer is simple: You make wise food choices by substituting one item for another.

But before we get to that, here are some other tips to consider about eating:

1 When you go out to eat have a healthy small snack beforehand—pretzels, half a bagel or half a banana. This will lessen the temptation of ordering everything on the menu by cutting hunger pangs. This is especially important if you go out to eat after your run, when hunger will be the highest and you'll be tempted to eat a lot of anything because you've "earned it."

2 Try to sit down and eat as soon as possible after your workouts. This makes sense because that is when your metabolism is the highest (so you'll burn more calories off) and because if you wait, that drives up hunger and slows down your metabolism (you will actually be hungrier, say, one hour after your run than half an hour later).

Now, some tips for cutting calories from your diet:

SUBSTITUTE	SAVE
mustard for mayonnaise	85 calories
water for soda pop	150 calories
skim milk for whole milk	90 calories per cup
pretzels for potato chips	50 calories per ounce
vanilla ice cream for Dove Bar	115 calories
yogurt for vanilla ice cream	85 calories
fig bar for brownie	50 calorie per cookie
egg whites for whole egg	59 calories per egg
regular pancakes for buttermilk	30 calorie per pancake
light beer for regular beer	30–79 calories per 8 fluid ounces

Day Twenty-nine Log

Time: _____

Place: _____

Comments: _____

_____

_____

20 MINUTES

Today's Run

Out 10 minutes, back 10 minutes.

Alcohol

▪ ▪ ▪ ▪ ▪ ▪ ▪ ▪ ▪ ▪ ▪ ▪ ▪

THE DANGER of using running in a weight-loss program is not injury or illness but feeling impervious—as if you're burning so many calories that you can eat and drink whatever you want and still lose weight.

Yes, running is replete with stories of great runners who lived on pizza for breakfast and many beers after their workouts. But these runners were different from you and me. As different as Shaquille O'Neal is from us. Genetically these people were born skinny, with large engines that enabled them to run 20 miles a day, barely breaking a sweat, and metabolism that burned like hell fire.

So unless you're made to spend two to three hours each day running, you've got to monitor your diet and another thing: watch your intake of alcohol.

Why is alcohol so bad for you when you're trying to lose weight? A bottle of beer or a glass of wine doesn't have many calories—150 to 250, about as much as a bagel. But alcohol is empty calories—there's no nutrition in them—and preferred calories, and that's where you run into trouble.

Empty calories do not refuel muscles after a hard run. And preferred calories mean that when alcohol hits your system, your metabolism immediately shifts its attention to burning that off, shunning other foods that might get packed on as fat later on—after your body has finished burning the alcohol and your metabolism has slowed down. Plus, you tend to eat more food when you are drinking alcohol because alcohol stimulates the appetite and lowers your inhibitions. Finally, alcohol is a diuretic. It makes you pee. That dehydrates you, sending your entire system out of whack.

So if you must drink, try a light beer or light wine. Limit yourself to one per day. Or cut your beer with ice, so you won't be dehydrating yourself in the process.

Day Thirty Log

Time: _____

Place: _____

Comments: _____

_____

_____

20 MINUTES

Today's Run

Out 10 minutes, back 10 minutes.

Where to Run

■ ■ ■ ■ ■ ■ ■ ■ ■ ■ ■ ■ ■

WHERE YOU run might be just as important as how much you run in your Run Away From Fat Program. If, for instance, you choose to run down a crowded sidewalk every day at 5:30 p.m., you'll soon give up the fight because of the hassle. But, if you find yourself traipsing through a park that Henry David Thoreau would call home, you'll keep at it day in and day out.

Therefore, let's look at the most popular training venues and see how they stack up against each other.

Neighborhood Streets and Sidewalks

They're good because you can go right outside your door—and finish at your door. Sidewalks can be bumpy and crowded, though, and streets can be dangerous (if you do run in the street always stick close to the side and run facing traffic, and if you are running at dusk or at night make sure to wear a reflective vest or reflective clothing). So pick a stretch of sidewalk that's not busy or a side street that no one ever uses. One trick that many runners use is running on the tree lawns between sidewalks and streets. This lessens the pounding on your knees from asphalt and concrete, but you have to watch your footing. Recommended only if you can't make other venues.

Golf Courses

These soft surfaces are ideal for beginning runners. Golf courses are fine early in the morning or late in the evening. On most public courses you can get away with running on the sides of the fairways (you might want to check first). But running through a golf course during peak hours can be dangerous. Otherwise it is a recommended surface.

Park Trails

Great running surfaces can be found at most parks. Many parks now have running and walking trails—as opposed to hiking trails, which can be bumpy and very hilly—that are perfect for running. Park trails offer the best of both worlds: a smooth surface and a serene setting. Highly recommended for all runs.

Open Fields

Open fields—like Little League baseball complexes or open city parks—can provide an interesting venue to run. Try running laps around them. Often this will take 5, 10, 15 minutes at one time. You just have to be careful of the footing. They're not manicured like park walking trails, and there can be ruts. Recommended for all runs.

Day Thirty-one Log

Time: _____

Place: _____

Comments: _____

_____

_____

15 MINUTES

Today's Run

Out 7 1/2 minutes, back 7 1/2 minutes.

Where to Run, Continued

Treadmills

A treadmill can give you a great running workout, if you can put up with the monotony. Therefore, treadmills are good for early in this program and on short days—10–15 minutes. Running for 30 minutes on a treadmill will often feel like hours, because you're going nowhere and looking at the same thing all the time. This might cause you to lose enthusiasm for running altogether, which is not what this program is about.

So if you do decide to run on a treadmill, try to pick a time at the health club when you have someone to talk to. At home, watch TV or listen to the stereo. The object is not to do a boring run. Treadmills are recommended for short runs. They're okay for long runs too, if you can tolerate it.

Outdoor Tracks

A good venue at almost any time because many times they're lighted and others are running as well. They also have solid footing. The one danger is lap counting, which might not seem too monotonous when you're just running for 10 or 15 minutes, but try going around in circles for a half hour and you'll know what I mean. The same goes double for indoor tracks—found at health clubs and colleges. They can be doubly monotonous because they're shorter. And they can also cause too much stress to your knees and hips (you are turning all the time).

Track etiquette says that slower runners move to the outside lanes of the track. This is good to know if you don't want to get plowed over by a sprinter. Recommended for short and intermediate runs.

Other Venues

The Beach

Fine if you can find hard-packed sand and an isolated stretch. But fluffy, sandy beaches made for beach towels and sun bathing are not good places to run. Your feet will sink too much, making running a chore. You will also get sand between your toes!

Stairways

This is a very good workout that you might try much later in your running career. Right now, as a beginner, hitting the stairs at lunch for, say, 10 minutes up (then ride the elevator back down) will beat your leg muscles to a pulp. If you make it all the way, you will be too tired and sore to run for the next couple of days.

For now keep these 3 things in mind when choosing a training venue:

1 Ease of access

2 Flatness

3 Safety

Day Thirty-two Log

Time: _____

Place: _____

Comments: _____

_____

_____

25 MINUTES

Today's Run

Out 12 1/2 minutes, back 12 1/2 minutes.
You've burned a lot of fat with your 20-minute runs. But you've also built endurance. Time to up the ante.

Increasing Time: 20–30 Minutes

T HE NEXT time block will take you from running for 20 minutes to 30 minutes—in two steps: 25 minutes first, then 30 minutes later.

Today is another big step for you—going from 20 minutes to 25 minutes. Twenty-five minutes is a good goal because you are fast approaching the time it will take you to run a 5K (3.1 miles). By racing a 5K every month or two, you will give your running program another goal and only add to your fat-burning capacity (but more on running a 5K later in this book).

Remember the basics for upping your time run (your long run) and you can't go wrong:

1 Make sure you are rested. (You ran just 15 minutes yesterday.)

2 Make sure you've had a high-carbohydrate snack.

3 Make sure you run on a flat, safe course.

④ Try to run with your training partner.

⑤ Start slowly for the first five minutes.

⑥ Enjoy yourself—you're running away from fat.

Day Thirty-three Log

Time: _____

Place: _____

Comments: _____

_____

_____

20 MINUTES

Today's Run

Out 10 minutes, back 10 minutes.

Dogs

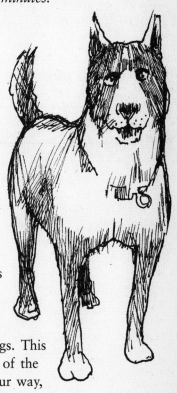

FOR SOME reason dogs— and some dog owners!—see runners as fair game. We are interrupting their walk, which they think, of course, is much more important than our run. And so we are the enemy.

Therefore, follow these rules to get your run in and keep Fido at bay.

1 If at all possible avoid dogs. This means run to the other side of the street when one stands in your way, or avoid a neighborhood or house where you have run into dogs before.

2 If you can't avoid them or come up on them unexpectedly, always speak at them in a calm, friendly voice. A startled dog can be an aggressive dog. Give the dog the right of way on a narrow pass—you don't want to challenge him.

3 If it growls or acts as if it is going to bite, stop. Face it and speak firmly. Go home. Or sit. Never take off and run. That's an invitation to a dog to chase you—and bite.

4 If you habitually encounter mean dogs, you might want to consider carrying pepper spray, or look for and pick up a big stick as you approach the area where you know dogs are lurking.

Day Thirty-four Log

Time: _____

Place: _____

Comments: _____

_____

_____

25 MINUTES

Today's Run

Out 12 1/2 minutes, back 12 1/2 minutes.

Testimonial

■ ■ ■ ■ ■ ■ ■ ■ ■ ■ ■ ■ ■

MEET SHELLEY. This 34-year-old businesswoman looks as if she just graduated from high school.

But don't tell her that. It would be an insult.

"After high school I weighed about 20 pounds more than I do now," she recalls. "And I was looking for something to help me lose some weight and get into a healthy lifestyle."

She found running. "Actually I tried other things first," she says. "I joined a health club and did aerobics and weight training and then eventually got into running on the treadmills."

She says she prefers running for two reasons. "The first is that you don't need a whole hour to get a good workout," she says. "I can get in some serious fat burning with just 20 minutes."

The second reason is that running is so accessible. "If I'm really crunched for time I won't drive to the club," she says, "I'll just lace up my shoes and get running out my front door."

Shelley now runs 4 or 5 days a week. She no longer has to worry about losing weight. "But now that I'm at my ideal weight, I find that running is the best way to maintain that weight," she says, with a laugh.

"Basically I do it now as a preventative measure."

Day Thirty-five Log

Time: _____

Place: _____

Comments: _____

_____

_____

0 MINUTES

Today's Run

0 minutes.

Soreness

W HEN YOU run, particularly early on in this program, you might encounter some soreness. I'm talking about tenderness in the leg muscles from running. This soreness in small doses is actually good. It means you are pushing your body more than it's used to, but it also means you are burning calories.

If you're used to only walking or you haven't been working out at all, soreness will not be uncommon in your first 10-minute runs (this program is set up for gradual increases in running to minimize the chances of muscle soreness). Soreness will strike not during your run but later on in the day or perhaps the next morning when you get out of bed.

Some of it might be stiffness—just an inactive body learning to be active again—like an engine that needs to go around a few times before it warms up. Stiffness will go away when you start moving and also if you incorporate a light stretching program (see Stretching, Days 46–54).

Soreness, on the other hand, will go away as you run more, but sometimes more running can cause more soreness. You need to be careful and follow these tips:

❶ If you have sore muscles take aspirin or ibuprofren after your run. It helps reduce the inflammation and speeds recovery.

❷ Also ice the affected area. A good way to ice is using an ice cup: paper cups of ice that you can peel back as they melt. Rub the sore muscle for 10 minutes with the ice cup using a circular motion.

❸ To help prevent soreness, don't run in worn-out shoes. Also run on soft surfaces as much as possible (grass, dirt trails). And work up the duration of your runs gradually. You might feel like jumping from 10 minutes to 30 minutes the next day, but you'll pay for it in soreness. And that soreness might be so severe that you'll end up skipping days. And not burning much fat.

❹ You might also try periodic massages—once a week—or self-massage. A home remedy is running cold water over your legs after your run—it helps flush out the muscles and prevents soreness.

As your body becomes more fit, soreness will gradually go away. It might not ever strike again. But if it does, you'll know what to do about it.

Day Thirty-six Log

Time: _____

Place: _____

Comments: _____

_____

_____

15 MINUTES

Today's Run

Out 7 1/2 minutes, back 7 1/2 minutes.

Variety: Don't Get in a Rut

T HERE ARE a few keys to completing this program: One is a good pair of shoes. Another is a running friend. A third is keeping the training interesting, and that's what I mean by variety.

Variety means not running in the same place at the same time every day.

1 We've already covered the best places to run. Now it's up to you to mix them up throughout the week. An easy way to do that is to assign venues to the days of the week. For example, run on a park trail Mondays, Wednesdays and Fridays. Run on a track Tuesdays and Thursdays. Get the picture?

2 Also, if you can, mix up the times that you run. Try the evenings on Monday, Wednesday and Friday. Lunchtime on Tuesday and Thursday. And early mornings on the weekends. (Of course, if you have an inflexible schedule, stick to the times when you know you can get in your run.)

You can also add variety to your workouts by doing one or two runs alone and two or three with your running friend. Weekends are also a good time to get together with a group, particularly later on in this program when you're running for more than 30 minutes.

Or make one day a week Fido's. Just make sure your dog is up to the challenge. Not all dogs are ready to go 30 minutes without stopping.

Or you can wear a Walkman on some runs. Many people find this helps with motivation. (Walkmans, however, should not be worn when you run on sidewalks or streets. You can't hear traffic—cars, dogs and pedestrians coming.)

And remember to save the best jokes for your runs with friends.

In summary, the whole idea is to make your run something to look forward to. Not something you begin to dread.

And that's the third key to help you Run Away From Fat.

Day Thirty-seven Log

Time: _____

Place: _____

Comments: _____

_____

_____

30 MINUTES

Today's Run

Out 15 minutes, back 15 minutes. You're bumping up your run by five minutes again, so start slowly.

Fat-Burning Workout #1: The Long Run

THE KEY workout for your Run Away From Fat Program is the long run. Veteran runners have long used the long run to increase endurance and burn off excess body fat, so why wouldn't you?

But before you fret about running for hours like a marathoner, let's state one thing first: The duration of your long run is relative to your fitness level. Any run that's longer than your average run at this point is a long run. This schedule is set up so that every two weeks or so you are going to be running longer than before. First 10 minutes, then 15 minutes, then 20 minutes, 30 minutes, and so on, working up to 40 minutes by the end of the 90 days.

Each time you bump up your time by five minutes this is your long run.

It is important to be well-rested for your long run and to get good rest after it. Your body will be reacting to the increased stress that an extra 5 minutes of running can put on it. (Remember: The way you get stronger so that you can burn more fat during your workouts is to stress your body, then rest it.)

Now to the long run. Long runs help you gain endurance—the ability to run farther—by stressing your heart and lungs and leg muscles. Long runs open capillaries in your legs to speed fuel to your muscles, and of course long runs help you to burn more fat as fuel. And the longer you run on your long run, the more you'll be able to run, and the more fat you will burn.

You'll increase your long run by no more than 5 minutes at a time. That's a good time increment spread out over 90 days because it ensures you will be building, not breaking down.

Remember to keep your pace slow on long runs. The goal is to run continuously for a certain amount of time, not to burn rubber. If you can't carry on a conversation while you're running, you're running too fast. This slow pace maximizes the percentage of fat that you burn as fuel and, over time according to some experts, you eventually teach the body to burn fat as the preferred fuel, over carbohydrates.

One final note on long runs: Since long runs are such great workouts and they burn gobs of fat, you might ask why don't I do them every day? Why don't I just run 2 hours today and every day thereafter?

Well, even Olympic marathoners don't do long runs more than twice a week. That's because they can't. Make no mistake about it: Long runs are stressful workouts. If you did them every day, you might get 4 or 5 days under your belt before you're injured or too tired to run for the next week.

Now get out and complete your 30-minute long run.

Day Thirty-eight Log

Time: _____

Place: _____

Comments: _____

_____

_____

20 MINUTES

Today's Run

Out for 10 minutes, back for 10 minutes.

Cold Weather

■ ■   ■   ■   ■   ■   ■   ■   ■   ■   ■   ■   ■

IF YOU'RE going to run outside in cold weather—and there really is not any reason why you shouldn't—then here are some tips.

1 Heed the cold but don't fear it: You can run when it's 40 degrees or 30 degrees, even in the low 20s. Anything lower than 20 degrees and you might want to head inside. A good guide is to have a windchill chart (see Day 40). A 30-degree day with a 15 mph head wind will feel like 9 degrees, so you should be prepared.

2 The best way to prepare to run in the cold is to dress in layers. And try to run out and back if you can. That is, start your run into the wind and finish your run with the wind at your back. That way, as you get further and further into your run, and a bit sweaty, you have the wind at your back, not in your face, so you won't chill.

3 Don't linger: The coldest part of your run is when you've finished. You're wet and cold. Go directly inside if you can and change clothes. If you can't—for example, you're at a trail-

head where you parked your car—immediately change into dry clothes over the top half of your body. New hat, shirt, and jacket. You will be cold at first, stripping off your sweaty clothes in the cold, but wet clothes do not insulate, and once you get past the first few seconds of cold, you will be dry and warm in no time.

4 Always cover your head: Forget about messing up your hair. Eighty percent of your body heat goes right out the top of your head when you run. There is no faster way to get a chill than running hatless.

5 Remember to drink: Though it won't be as obvious at first, you will sweat in 30 degree weather. Your body has lost fluid and it needs to be replaced. Your mouth just won't be as parched as it will be on a hot summer day. Have fluid ready at the end of your run. You might want to make up a thermos of hot water or lemonade to warm you up instantly.

Day Thirty-nine Log

Time: _____

Place: _____

Comments: _____

_____

_____

30 MINUTES

Today's Run

Out for 15 minutes, back for 15 minutes.

Windchill

∎ ∎ ∎ ∎ ∎ ∎ ∎ ∎ ∎ ∎ ∎ ∎

W ON'T I freeze my lungs if I run outside in cold weather?

That's the question every nonrunner has asked before putting one foot out the door in winter.

The simple answer is no. Think of all the skaters, skiers, kids on sleds working up a sweat, breathing deeply all that cold potentially lung-freezing air, and you see how ridiculous that question is.

That said, there is something you need to look out for when running outside in the cold—and that is windchill.

A strong wind on a 40 degree day can make it feel like 20. The wind actually takes heat from your body. So be prepared and take precautions when the wind is up.

Also consult this windchill chart.

WINDCHILL CHART

WIND SPEED (MPH)	THERMOMETER READING (°F)							
	50	40	30	20	10	0	-10	-20
Calm	50	40	30	20	10	0	-10	-20
5	48	37	27	16	6	-5	-15	-26
10	40	28	16	4	-9	-24	-33	-46
15	36	22	9	-5	-18	-32	-45	-58
20	32	18	4	-10	-25	-39	-52	-67
25	30	16	0	-15	-29	-44	-59	-74
30	28	13	-2	-18	-33	-48	-63	-79
35	27	11	-4	-20	-35	-51	-67	-82
40	26	10	-6	-21	-37	-53	-69	-85

LITTLE DANGER (for properly clothed person)	INCREASING DANGER (exposed flesh may freeze)	GREAT DANGER (flesh may freeze within 3 min.)

Day Forty Log

Time: _____

Place: _____

Comments: _____

_____

_____

25 MINUTES

Today's Run

Out for 12 1/2 minutes, back for 12 1/2 minutes.

Running In the Heat

A SIMPLE rule for running in severe heat (anything that feels very uncomfortable: it could be 82 degrees and very humid or 95 degrees and sunny) is this: Don't.

If you don't have to, don't do it. You won't, as you have learned, lose more weight by sweating more. You're more likely to get dehydrated and pass out from lack of fluids or put yourself at risk for heat-related injuries. (Generally, any run when the temperature is over 80 degrees should be approached with care. Do it wisely.)

To avoid running in severe heat, run early in the morning or late in the evening. Or run inside in air-conditioned comfort if that is an option for you.

If you do run outside in the heat, make sure you dress in loose-fitting clothing (a T-shirt and a pair of shorts is enough) and run on a shaded route, say, through a wooded trail. If you have to run in the sun, make sure you wear a hat—a ball cap will suffice, as long as it's not wool.

Drink plenty of water before (16 ounces) and after you run (16 ounces for each 15 minutes). And during your run if that's possible.

Try this for today to simulate a heat run: Drink water at the start. Now run for 5 minutes and turn around. When you get back to the start at 10 minutes, take another drink. Now run out for 5 more minutes and turn around.

When you've finished, you've run 20 minutes in the heat and you've had water at the halfway point, beginning and end.

That's a smart way to run in the heat.

Day Forty-one Log

Time: _____

Place: _____

Comments: _____

_____

_____

30 MINUTES

Today's Run

Out 15 minutes, back 15 minutes.

Testimonial

· · · · · · · · · · · · · · ·

MEET TIM. He's a 36-year-old businessman who also happens to be a former collegiate distance runner—and a very good one at that.

But like many athletes in college, he spent the years directly after college without much activity. "I led the typical sedentary lifestyle," Tim recalls. "I had always been a big eater, but when I ran, it didn't matter. But as soon as I stopped running, boy, did it begin to matter."

That first year after college, Tim put on 20 pounds. After a few more years he packed on another 18.

One day he looked at himself. Not quite 30 but going on 50. "I decided to get back into running again," he says.

The weight came off quickly, so that today he's just a few pounds over his college weight. "I don't run the miles I did in college, maybe 20–30 a week," he says. "But the key thing for me is to keep the running constant: Get in four or five days a week and don't take weeks off at a time. If I do that, my weight is fine."

He also realized he'd missed his old friend—running. "On the days that I run I feel better all the way around," he says. "If, for instance, I have a bad day at the office, then I go for a run, and I don't feel bad at all by the time I get home."

Day Forty-two Log

Time: _____

Place: _____

Comments: _____

_____

_____

0 MINUTES

Today's Run

0 minutes.

Heed Heat Injuries

■ ■ ■ ■ ■ ■ ■ ■ ■ ■ ■ ■ ■ ■ ■

YOU SHOULD know the warning signs of heat-related injuries. They progress through three phases: 1) heat cramps, 2) heat exhaustion, 3) heat stroke.

1 Heat cramps are cramps in the leg muscles. They are the most common and least serious of the three. They are caused by intense sweating and the loss of minerals (sodium and potassium) that results. If you get heat cramps, stop and walk and try to drink or eat foods that put back these minerals into your body, such as bananas or Gatorade. (Eating a banana a day will help ward off heat cramps.)

2 Heat exhaustion means that you are experiencing weakness, dizzy spells, goose bumps and a rapid heart rate. You're seriously dehydrated, and your heart is stressed to its limit. If you experience heat exhaustion, stop and get out of the sun and drink plenty of fluids immediately, or else you might get heat stroke.

3 Heat stroke is the most serious. Your body stops sweating, and your temperature climbs. Confusion and slurred speech follow, and you may pass out. At this point the body must be cooled to protect against tissue damage or possibly death. People who have survived heat stroke are more prone to heat injuries because heat stroke has thrown their internal heat regulators out of whack.

The key with heat-related injuries is to heed the warning signs of heat cramps, and you should never have to worry about heat exhaustion or heat stroke.

Day Forty-three Log

Time: _____

Place: _____

Comments: _____

_____

_____

30 MINUTES

Today's Run

Out 15 minutes, back 15 minutes.

Warmup

A GOOD warmup is key to every run. Over time you will learn to develop a warmup routine of your own. A warmup gets you ready to run, like warming up your car in the morning. You wouldn't just jump into a cold car and take off at high speeds down the road, would you?

A warmup can consist of a little or a lot. Again, learn to do what you are comfortable with. A little warmup might be simply walking the first 30 seconds of every run. That way you ease into your run so it is not so much of a shock to your body. (You should always start every run walking or at least running very, very slowly. Never run fast at the beginning of your run. That could cause injury like a pulled muscle or make the rest of your run seem too hard—because you are already out of breath.)

What other things can you do to warm up? A little light stretching is fine. Circle your arms, twist your trunk. Anything to get the kinks out and the blood circulating more rapidly.

If you work 9–5 and know that you'll be running at 5:30, you might want to sneak in a few stretches at 4:45 or take the stairs at that time or practice lifting your knees at your desk. That could be part of your warmup routine.

Other than the physical, there are mental aspects to warming up. You might want to stand still and take 10 relaxed breaths before you begin your run. Clear you mind. And envision the run ahead.

Okay, ready? Now warm up and then go out and run off the fat.

Day Forty-four Log

Time: _____

Place: _____

Comments: _____
_____
_____

30 MINUTES

Today's Run

Out 15 minutes, back 15 minutes.

Cooldown

▪ ▪ ▪ ▪ ▪ ▪ ▪ ▪ ▪ ▪ ▪ ▪

JUST AS important as the warmup is the cooldown. Again, it can be as brief as walking for 30 seconds, or it can take up 10 minutes or so.

What you are doing with your cooldown is gradually revving your engine down (You wouldn't cut the engine on your car going 50 mph down the road, would you?). The cooldown starts near the end of your run and really is a preparation for your run the following day. By flushing the system of waste products built up during your run, the cooldown helps prevent stiff muscles for the next day.

While many runners might be tempted to sprint the last 50 yards of their run, you should actually be slowing down at that point, making your cadence slower and slower and slower, until you get to the point where you walk. (Never just stop cold. That will cause waste products to pool in your legs.)

While walking shake out your arms and take a few deep breaths. You should walk for at least a minute, preferably 2–3 minutes or more. After walking you can stop and perform some gentle stretches. The key is to find a cooldown that works for you and stick to it.

In no time you'll be doing your cooldown by rote, without even thinking about it.

Other options for cooldown: You might want to grab your water bottle and walk with it, sipping fluid. (A mental key to walking your cooldown is to turn back and walk the way you came. Don't ask me why, but this is mentally refreshing. Something about retracing your steps seems to work on the psyche. Also, knowing that you've already covered this ground or stretch of track feels good.)

As you progress in your Run Away From Fat Program and your endurance is up, you might want to add sit-ups and pushups or even light weight training to your cooldown routines two times a week (more on this later).

The whole idea of the cooldown is to physically and mentally wind down so you'll be primed for tomorrow's run.

Day Forty-five Log

Time: _____

Place: _____

Comments: _____

_____

_____

25 MINUTES

Today's Run

Out 12 1/2 minutes, back 12 1/2 minutes.

Stretch It Out

I F STRETCHING isn't a part of your running program, it should be. As you run longer and more frequently, stiffness becomes a possibility, and one way to help prevent stiffness (and any more severe injury in general) is by stretching.

Stretching enables you to have the smoothest run possible, sort of like adding oil to the gear shaft of your car's engine.

You can stretch for 2 or 20 minutes. Every day or 3 times a week. The important thing is to do some stretching, rather than none at all.

Some basic rules for stretching:

1 Never stretch a cold muscle. If you're running early in the morning, never get out of bed and stretch—you're only setting yourself up to strain a muscle. The best time to stretch is after your run, when your body is cooling down.

2 Never stretch a sore muscle. Sore muscles mean you have small tears (microtears) in the muscle fiber. By stretching you are just ripping them open further. Wait till soreness subsides before you stretch again.

③ Stretch to the point of mild uncomfortableness—not strain or pain. A stretching program, like this running program, should work with gradual increases, stretching a little bit, then a little bit more a week later, to increases flexibility. If you try for too hard a stretch the first time out, you are going to tear a muscle.

④ Don't bounce when you stretch. Hold each stretch for five seconds to start, then work up each week by 5 seconds more until you reach 30 seconds. Muscle fibers learn to stretch by constant stretching over time. Not by jerking down and then back up.

There are a variety of stretches, but the seven key stretches on the following pages can form a good core workout for anyone in this program. Just give yourself a few minutes to cooldown after your run, then find a comfortable spot to stretch it out.

Day Forty-six Log

Time: _____

Place: _____

Comments: _____

_____

_____

30 MINUTES

Today's Run

Out 15 minutes, back 15 minutes.

Calf Stretch

■ ■ ■ ■ ■ ■ ■ ■ ■ ■ ■ ■ ■

THE CALF muscle is the major muscle in the back of your leg between your foot and your knee.

The Stretch

Stand two feet from a wall. Place both palms on the wall for support. Bend your left leg and lean toward the wall, keeping your right knee straight. Hold the stretch for 5 seconds. You should feel a stretch in the right calf. If you don't, move your feet further from the wall and lean in and try it again. Repeat for the other leg.

Day Forty-seven Log

Time: _____

Place: _____

Comments: _____

_____

_____

Today's Run

Out 15 minutes, back 15 minutes.

Quadriceps Stretch

Y OUR QUADRICEPS is the large muscle in the front of your thigh.

The Stretch

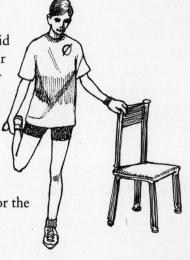

Stand next to a chair or solid object and with your left leg near the object. Balance yourself by grasping the object with your left hand. With your right hand reach behind you and grab your ankle. Slowly raise your ankle toward your butt until you feel a stretch in the quadriceps. Hold for three seconds. Reverse for the left quadriceps.

Day Forty-eight Log

Time: _____

Place: _____

Comments: _____

_____

_____

30 MINUTES

Today's Run

Out 15 minutes, back 15 minutes. Remember: The goal is to run for 30 minutes. Don't worry about speed.

Testimonial

MEET DAVE.
A few years ago this 54-year-old airline pilot started on a running program as a way to get back in the cockpit following a double bypass operation on his heart.

"I knew after the operation I had to make some changes in my life," he says. "I wasn't grossly overweight but I had packed on about 20 pounds. I guess you could say I was your typical middle-aged slob. I ate a lot of red meat and eggs. Exercise for me was a game of softball or going water skiing. I had no endurance at all."

Dave cleaned up his diet, and at the same time he laced up a pair of new running shoes. "My first run was just a few minutes," he recalls. "But I was determined to stick with it."

The runs became gradually longer, and the weight started melting off his frame—more than 20 pounds of it.

Eventually he was fit enough to return to his job. "The FAA said if I could run 20 miles at a time, I could climb up the stairs to the cockpit," he says.

Today Dave uses running to keep his weight steady and maintain an active lifestyle. "I actually have more energy now than I did 30 years ago," he says. "And it's the running that has done it."

Day Forty-nine Log

Time: _____

Place: _____

Comments: _____

_____

_____

30 MINUTES

Today's Run

Out for 15 minutes, back for 15 minutes.

Hamstring Stretch

■ ■ ■ ■ ■ ■ ■ ■ ■ ■ ■ ■ ■ ■ ■ ■

THE HAMSTRING is the large muscle that runs along the back of the thigh.

The Stretch

Find a stool or bench 6–12 inches off the ground. Steady yourself, and then raise your right foot onto the bench. Bend your left knee for added balance, but keep your right knee straight and lean toward your right foot by bending forward from the waist, keeping your back straight. You should feel a stretch in your right hamstring. Hold for three seconds. Switch legs to stretch the left hamstring.

Day Fifty Log

Time: _____

Place: _____

Comments: _____

_____

_____

30 MINUTES

Today's Run

15 minutes out, 15 minutes back.

Back Stretch

· · · · · · · · · · · · · ·

YOUR BACK plays a major role in running fitness. A bad back will keep you from running for days and maybe weeks.

The Stretch

Stand upright with your back straight and your stomach tight. Inhale, then slowly raise both hands over your head until they touch above your head. You should feel a stretch throughout your back. Hold for three seconds, then exhale and bring your arms down slowly.

Day Fifty-one Log

Time: _____

Place: _____

Comments: _____

_____

_____

25 MINUTES

Today's Run

Out 12 1/2 minutes, back 12 1/2 minutes.

Groin Stretch

■ ■ ■ ■ ■ ■ ■ ■ ■ ■ ■ ■ ■ ■ ■

T HE GROIN area is an oft-neglected part of your legs, but a crucial one that needs to be stretched for you to maximize your stride.

The Stretch

Sit on the floor with the soles of your feet pressed close together or as close as you can get them. Lean forward, keeping your back straight, and hold for 5 seconds.

Day Fifty-two Log

Time: _____

Place: _____

Comments: _____

_____

_____

30 MINUTES

Today's Run

Out 15 minutes, back 15 minutes.

Side Stretch

OVERALL A very good stretch that loosens up your torso and helps you run more smoothly.

The Stretch

Standing with your feet shoulder-width apart and knees slightly bent, slowly bend to the right side and bring your left arm over your head. Hold for five seconds. Repeat on the other side.

Day Fifty-three Log

Time: _____

Place: _____

Comments: _____

_____

_____

30 MINUTES

Today's Run

Out 15 minutes, back 15 minutes.

Hip and Buttocks Stretch

· ·

LOOSE HIPS will help your running economy—you'll cover more ground with less effort. The same goes for the buttocks.

The Stretch

Sit on the floor with your left leg straight. Bend your right knee and cross it over your left thigh, placing your right foot flat on the floor along the outside of your left knee. Place your left elbow on the outside of your right knee. Slowly twist to the right, applying force to the right knee. Hold for five seconds. Repeat on the other side.

Day Fifty-four Log

Time: _____

Place: _____

Comments: _____

_____

_____

30 MINUTES

Today's Run

Out 15 minutes, back 15 minutes.

Hand and Ankle Weights

■ ■ ■ ■ ■ ■ ■ ■ ■ ■ ■ ■ ■ ■ ■ ■ ■

IF YOU were a walker or have seen a lot of walkers, you know what hand and ankle weights are.

Hand weights are small enough to be clutched in your hands. You pump them vigorously when you walk, adding a strength workout to your walk.

Ankle weights are strapped around your ankles and are designed to firm the leg muscles by putting more weight on your legs.

Don't use them.

They are bad for running. First of all, clutching hand weights while you are running is dangerous. When you run, you swing your arms faster than when you walk, and this might cause you to drop the weights on your foot. You might even throw them accidentally and hit someone else. Second, if you start running with hand weights, you're more likely to stop sooner in your run. You'll finish a 15-minute run with sore arms, but that won't do you any good if you were scheduled to run for 25 minutes. You won't burn much fat. Sore arms burn very few extra calories. (And, ladies, if you're worried about the wattle under your arm, the best way to get rid of it is to burn more fat by running more.)

Ankle weights won't fly off your feet, but they will cause you to cut short your run from fatigue. Plus, it's not just the muscles that get fatigued. Ankle weights can put severe stress on your knees and hips, and that can cause ligament damage in those areas. There's no faster way to cut short a running program than getting injured knees and hips.

Day Fifty-five Log

Time: _____

Place: _____

Comments: _____

_____

_____

20 MINUTES

Today's Run

Out 10 minutes, back 10 minutes.

Testimonial

■ ■ ■ ■ ■ ■ ■ ■ ■ ■ ■ ■ ■ ■ ■

Meet Chris. She's an attractive, 34-year-old substitute schoolteacher.

That means the morning hours are filled with anticipation and trepidation.

Will the phone ring, telling her she has 45 minutes to get to a certain school to teach? Or will it stay silent, meaning she can stay in bed?

Not quite.

"If I don't have to teach that day, I start planning when I can run," she says.

Chris estimates that she has lost 15 pounds running over the years.

"I'm not hard-core," she says. "But I get out three or four times a week." She pauses. "I have to," she laughs. "Because I'm not 19 years old anymore, and I have learned that if I don't stay active, the weight comes back on that much faster."

Chris knows that running plus a healthy diet is the best way to lose weight or maintain the weight loss than you have achieved.

"Running keeps the metabolism going," she says. "But then it's up to you not to eat the wrong things. Don't load up on beer or fatty foods. But the nice thing about running regularly is that when you are on a running program, you tend to not want to eat those kinds of foods, because your body starts to crave healthy foods to fuel it after your run."

Day Fifty-six Log

Time: _____

Place: _____

Comments: _____

_____

_____

0 MINUTES

Today's Run

0 minutes.

Join a Group

YOU'VE RUN for almost two months!
You've probably dropped some weight, and you feel pretty good. This running stuff, you say to yourself, might be for you.

One of the goals of this book is to help you incorporate running into your lifestyle, not only to lose weight in 90 days but also give you continued fitness, energy, weight loss and fun for the rest of your life.

One of the best ways of continuing to run is to join a group.

Wherever you live you probably have a running group close by. True, you may have seen groups of very fast and very fit men and women blowing by you on the path or track or street, but running groups include runners of all abilities.

The first step is to find out about running clubs in your area. If you don't have a clue, contact the Road Runners Club of America for assistance (visit their website at www.rrca.org to find a club in your area). Find the club closest to you and give them a call. Most clubs have monthly meetings where you can become acquainted with other runners—many of your ability. During these meetings you can learn about your new sport from guest speakers and also arrange group runs. Many clubs offer a weekend group run on a Saturday morning—usually the weekly long run—and then a midweek run of lesser distance but greater intensity. Show up and find out what these are like. You won't make it the full distance, but you can start with them and then do your own workout and meet them for dinner or breakfast afterward.

In addition, most clubs publish monthly newsletters and even a phone directory, so you can keep up on club news and have someone you can call when you want to meet for a run.

Spend your rest day looking up information on running clubs around you.

Day Fifty-seven Log

Time: _____

Place: _____

Comments: _____

_____

_____

20 MINUTES/ STRIDES

Today's Run

Out for 10 minutes, and on the way back run 2 x 5 strides at a faster pace. Make sure to run easily for three minutes between each set of five strides.

Intensity

Y OU'VE LEARNED the meaning of duration in running, upping your runs to 10 minutes, 15 minutes, 20 minutes, 30 minutes and 35 minutes.

Now let's get acquainted with another aspect of running that will help you burn fat and lose weight: intensity.

The root word is *intense*. But don't let that scare you away.

Intensity is just a way of saying that you are going to work a little harder than you would on your average runs. By adding intensity to your run, you burn more fat in less time—because your metabolism is cranked up higher—and you also give yourself a break from running the same speed and duration most other days. It's something different.

In short, intensity burns fat and keep you interested at the same time.

Examples of intense workouts are hills, pickups and tempo runs, all of which I will cover soon. But for now you can practice running today, say for 5 seconds, at a little bit faster pace than usual.

How do you do that?

For starters, lower your arms a bit. Lean forward slightly. And concentrate on picking up your legs more quickly off the ground. Lift your knees, but not too high. You want to get your legs off the ground, in the air, and back on the ground, faster than you normally do.

This is called turnover.

Run for 5 strides at a more intense pace. It's just a little faster than your normal pace.

Now you're getting the hang of it.

Run for 3 minutes more at your normal pace and try running faster for 5 strides again.

You'll find yourself breathing harder, perhaps panting a little. Your heart will be beating faster, too.

That's okay. That means you're working harder and burning more fat and calories in the process.

This will give you a taste of what you'll be trying the week after.

Hills.

Day Fifty-eight Log

Time: _____

Place: _____

Comments: _____

_____

_____

15 MINUTES

Today's Run

Out for 7 1/2 minutes, back for 7 1/2 minutes. This 15-minute run will help your legs recover from yesterday's strides.

The Best Time to Run

T HE BEST time to run is, of course, the time you can fit it into your schedule. For some, that means getting up an hour earlier each morning to fit in a 30-minute run. Others might hop outside during their lunch hour to run or run late at night when the rest of the family has gone to bed.

If it is at all possible, the best time to run is in the evening—at the end of the day. Evening runs are preferable for several reasons:

1 You don't have to rush to go to work afterward, enabling you to enjoy your workout and cooldown more. You can also get in a good stretching routine afterward, or do calisthenics or weights.

2 It gives you something to look forward to during the day. Stare at the clock: It's 2:10 p.m., 10 minutes later than the last time you looked. But if you're running at 5:30 after work in the park, the office job might not seem so bad.

③ It relaxes you. And gets you ready for a nice evening. If you've never done an evening run and then gone out to dinner, you won't understand the glow that accompanies you—inside and out.

④ It's closest to the biggest meal of the day—dinner. And you're more apt to burn it off because your metabolism is cranked from your run.

So run in the evening, if you can. You'll thank yourself.

Day Fifty-nine Log

Time: _____

Place: _____

Comments: _____

_____

_____

25 MINUTES

Today's Run

Out for 12 1/2 minutes, back for 12 1/2 minutes.

Consistency Is the Key

S OME DAYS you just can't squeeze in a run no matter how you juggle your schedule.

This is okay. As long as you it doesn't become a habit. And as long as you don't miss two days in a row . . . and then try and double your next run to make up for those lost days.

Consistency is the key to this and every other exercise program. You need to run regularly to regularly burn fat and calories and build strength. Missing days interrupts that steady burn and also tempts you to do too much when you get back on track—which can lead to injury or illness.

Follow this program as faithfully as you can. It's designed to keep you consistent without wearing you out. Try to follow each workout as closely as possible (or incorporate the five-minute rule). If you do miss days, don't panic and add extra time to your next run. Always remember that five steady consistent workouts a week are much better than two hard ones.

For example, if you ran 50 minutes Monday and then 50 minutes again Tuesday, you would burn roughly 1,000 calories. But then if you were too tired and sore to run for the next three days, that would be it.

But, on the other hand, if you ran 30–35 minutes each of those days, you would burn more than 1,500 calories.

See what I mean?

Consistency is the key to weight loss. Consistency is the key to fitness. Consistency is the key to the rest of your life.

Day Sixty Log

Time: _____

Place: _____

Comments: _____

_____

_____

30 MINUTES

Today's Run

15 minutes out, 15 minutes back.

Weight Training

As a supplement to your Run Away From Fat Program, I've suggested push-ups and sit-ups. But if you really want to increase the caloric burn, you should try some weight training.

"Now, wait a minute," you may be thinking, "you want me to pump iron like Arnold? My legs are big enough already, thank you." First of all, I don't want you to pump iron like Arnold. And second of all, you won't increase the size of your legs, just tone your muscle. All we're asking for is 20 minutes 2 times a week.

These workouts can be done with hand weights, a home gym or Nautilus machines at a health club (see a personal trainer at a gym if you have questions about the machines). What you want to shoot for is 12 repetitions of each lift. At the beginning, try to find a weight for each lift that you can lift comfortably 12 times. Week by week increase the weight by 5 pounds or 10 pounds until you get to the point where you have to work to get numbers 8–12 done. Stay with that weight until number 12 becomes easy again; then increase the weight. You are getting stronger.

When you lift each weight, count to 2 on the way up and 4 on the way down. This maximizes your muscle workout.

If you have never lifted weights before, you might be a little stiff the next day. This is normal. Just make sure you don't lift again until at least 3 days later. For example, if you lifted on Monday, make your next weight workout no sooner than Thursday.

A good time to do your weight workout is after your run. That way, you'll continue to burn fat at a high rate because your metabolism is stoked from your run. (If you try to lift weights before you run, you risk being stiff and not completing your run.)

Here's a list of the lifts for simple 2-times-a-week weight training:

Biceps Curl: Targets your biceps muscles and forearms.
Triceps Extension: Targets your triceps.
Lat Pulldown: Targets back and shoulders.
Bench Press: Targets your chest and shoulders.
Leg Curl: Targets your glutes and hamstrings.
Leg Extension: Targets quadriceps muscles in your thighs.

So after your run today, try to incorporate a light weight workout. Once it becomes part of your routine—say, every Monday and Thursday—it won't take much time at all.

Day Sixty-one Log

Time: _____

Place: _____

Comments: _____

_____

_____

15 MINUTES

Today's Run

7 1/2 minutes out, 7 1/2 minutes back.

Fun

THE GOAL of this program is to keep you running way past the 90 days in this book.

And the best way to do this is to keep running fun.

When you first started this program, the last thing you thought running would be was fun. It was something you had to do because you wanted to lose weight and body fat. But, by now, you're beginning to see what we mean by fun.

Here're some tips for keeping running fun:

1. Always start with a warmup walk, working into a slow jog, then the pace you want to run for today.

2. Try not to run in the same place three days in a row.

3. Reward yourself after hard runs—faster or longer efforts— by going out for healthy meals afterward.

4. Run with a training partner.

5 Run with a group.

6 Don't stare at your watch.

7 Enjoy nature. On nice days run in the park.

8 Don't forget Fido. If your dog is a runner, take him along.

9 Say "Hi" to fellow runners and walkers.

10 Cool down. Remember to walk and stretch after each run. This helps you wind down and makes tomorrow's run easier, too, because it cleans lactic acid from your muscles.

Day Sixty-two Log

Time: _____

Place: _____

Comments: _____

_____

_____

30 MINUTES

Today's Run

15 minutes out, 15 minutes back.

Testimonial

MEET CHRISTINE. She's a 27-year-old Ph.D. student in psychology.

That, of course, means that for the past few years she spent a lot of time hitting the books at all hours of the day and night. And because of this school-imposed sedentary lifestyle, she'd gained a few more pounds than she would have liked.

So she decided to do something about it.

"I tried aerobics at first," she says. "I went to class three times a week and did all the routines. I found that aerobics did some good for toning my muscles, but when I got on the scale I didn't see much weight coming off."

So she started running. Just 3 to 4 days a week—20–40 minutes a day.

"It was amazing," she says. "I lost 4 pounds that first month."

She continued running and lost the weight she'd set out to get rid of. And then she found she was hooked.

"Running, I found, was the best way to lose weight," she says. "But I also found that it was the most worthwhile exercise for me because of my schedule. I could do it anytime and pick up the pace if I wanted to or slow it down if I chose to. Sometimes I would finish so out of breath that I couldn't talk.

"But that sure makes it feel good when I am done."

Day Sixty-three Log

Time: _____

Place: _____

Comments: _____

_____

_____

0 MINUTES

Today's Run

0 minutes.

Plan a Running Weekend Getaway

▪ ▪ ▪ ▪ ▪ ▪ ▪ ▪ ▪ ▪ ▪ ▪ ▪ ▪ ▪ ▪

Y OU'VE BEEN running now for nine weeks. You've covered
more than 30 minutes in one run. Now's the time to go for a
weekend running getaway.

You have two options:

1 Pick a nice locale that features a great trail or scenic road to
run on the weekend. Perhaps there is a great national park that
you've always wanted to go to. Or a certain spot at the beach
beckons. Book yourself a hotel room with your running
friends or significant other (who should be running by now,
too). Drive or make the short flight on Friday. Have a relaxing
evening while you plan your morning run. Get up and run 35
minutes in the morning; then have brunch and sightsee the rest
of the day.

The next morning go for another run in a place you spot-
ted yesterday afternoon. After brunch and more sightseeing,
head on home.

2 If you don't want to travel far, leave home on a Saturday
morning and drive a few hours to your destination, say, a na-

tional park. Get out and run, and then spend the rest of the day sightseeing before you return home.

This change in locale is very important to your Run Away From Fat Program. You will be celebrating over two months of running, and this "special run" will reinvigorate your training.

When you get back home you will find you can do your usual runs with renewed enthusiasm.

Day Sixty-four Log

Time: _____

Place: _____

Comments: _____

_____

_____

20 MINUTES/
HILLS

Today's Run

Jog for 5 minutes around the base of a slight hill, run 5 times up the hill, resting one minute. After you get back to the bottom, jog five minutes.

Fat-Burning Workout Number #2:
Be Bully on Hills

A GOOD fat-burning workout is to run on hills. For this workout find a short hill (30 to 50 yards) that isn't so steep that you have to walk up but is steep enough that if you run it, your heart rate increases and you breathe harder, too.

Warm up by jogging for 5 minutes before you get to the hill. Then you're going to run up it and jog back down. Try for three times, making sure to catch your breath before you begin again. Complete your workout by jogging for 5 minutes to cool down.

Hills act as great fat burners and also transitional workouts from slow jogging to faster running (which also burns more calories). Going up hills, you'll feel your heart pump hard—perhaps in your temple. That means your body is working harder, and you're burning more calories for fuel. Hills, if done wisely, will make you stronger (making everyday runs seem easier) and even shape up some trouble spots (they're a great toner for the legs and butt).

Here are some tricks to running hills:

1 Ease into them. Gradually pick up the pace on the flat before you reach the hill.

2 Lower your arms. When you start going up, lower your arms below your waist and pump them more.

3 Lift your knees.

4 Lean into the hill. Trying to remain straight backed will cause you to slow down because gravity is working against you, pulling you back.

5 Try to establish a smooth, controlled stride. Get into a rhythm and keep it all the way to the top.

You should arrive at the top slightly winded, but not exhausted. If you bend over and gasp for breath, either the hill is too steep or too long, or you ran too fast.

If you are gasping for breath, find another hill or slow down. You should finish this workout feeling tired, but not so exhausted that you can't get out of bed the next morning and run.

Day Sixty-five Log

Time: _____

Place: _____

Comments: _____

_____

_____

15 MINUTES

Today's Run

7 1/2 minutes out, 7 1/2 minutes back.

The Dreaded Side Stitch

■ ■ ■ ■ ■ ■ ■ ■ ■ ■ ■ ■ ■ ■ ■ ■

ALL RUNNERS encounter the side stitch periodically, but beginning runners are more prone to them because, first of all, they aren't as fit as those who have been running for a couple of months or several years. Second, they don't know how to prevent side stitches, which is the real key to dealing with this annoying pain in the side.

First of all, what is a side stitch? It's actually more of a cramp, and it can strike either on the right side of your stomach below the rib cage or on the left side. It can come on slowly, building until you can't take it anymore. Or it can strike suddenly; it feels so painful that you are reduced to a slow walk or sitting on a bench.

Side stitches are caused by two things. The left side stitch generally is a food cramp. You've eaten too much too close to your run, and the food is not digested and is causing a cramp. To prevent this, make sure to eat your last meal at least 2 hours before your run. (All runners will vary. Some can get away with a snack an hour before a run. Others need a full 3 hours to let all food digest. Learn your own limits.)

A left side stitch is hard to get rid of once it strikes. You may have to slow down or walk the rest of your run.

The right side stitch is more common, and more painful. It is sometimes called a diaphragm cramp and is caused by not warming up enough. Morning runners, who hop out of bed and hit the road, invariably encounter right side stitches more than others. But just because you run in the evening does not mean you won't get a right side stitch too. If you skip your warmup, you're more prone to a right side stitch. Also if you pick up the pace suddenly rather than gradually, you're more prone to a right side stitch.

Anything that forces the diaphragm—what moves up and down with your lungs when you breathe—to suddenly shift gears can cause a right side stitch.

I'll explain how to get rid of the right side stitch on Day 67.

Day Sixty-six Log

Time: _____

Place: _____

Comments: _____

_____

_____

25 MINUTES

Today's Run

12 1/2 minutes out, 12 1/2 minutes back.

Getting Rid of a Side Stitch

■ ■ ■ ■ ■ ■ ■ ■ ■ ■ ■ ■ ■ ■ ■ ■

To PREVENT a right side stitch, you must take your warmup seriously. That means beginning each run with a slow jog for at least five minute before, if so desired, picking up the pace—and picking up the pace gradually.

You might also want to practice belly breathing before you begin your run, to loosen up the diaphragm. Belly breathing means that you are inflating both lungs to their fullest and stretching the diaphragm likewise. To belly breathe put your hands on your belly when you inhale and try to fill your lungs all the way to the bottom—which will force the belly to rise—hold it, then exhale slowly. Do this 10 times before you begin your warmup if you are prone to right side stitches.

If a right side stitch strikes when you run, slow down and lean into the stitch, breathing deeply. If this doesn't alleviate it, stop and bend over on that side, gently massaging the area. Try walking for a few minutes while belly breathing. Gradually pick up the pace to a jog. If the stitch still doesn't go away, walk the rest of the run. Forcing yourself to run through a painful right side stitch can actually cause a cramp that could linger for days, keeping you from running the rest of the week.

Remember, prevention is the key for this annoying malady.

Make sure you eat well before you run and that you warm up well, and you shouldn't have a problem.

If you don't do these things, expect running to become a pain in the side.

Day Sixty-seven Log

Time: _____

Place: _____

Comments: _____

_____

_____

35 MINUTES

Today's Run

17 1/2 minutes out, 17 1/2 minutes back.

Increase Time: 30–40 Minutes

O VER THE last few weeks you've worked up to where you can run 30 minutes without stopping.

Now the next step, upping that run to 40 minutes. (Plus, 40 minutes is a good goal because it not only boosts the number of calories and the amount of fat you are burning, but at 40 minutes you start to maximize your aerobic fitness; that is, your heart and lungs adapt to this time and become stronger and more fit.)

We're going to work up to 40 minutes in two steps. Remember, you don't have to run faster, just run for 5 minutes longer. We'll target today as one to increase your running time. Once you have reached 35 one day a week, try to run another day at 35 minutes.

Okay, let's get busy.

Instead of running 15 minutes out and then 15 minutes back, you are going to run 17½ minutes out and 17½ minutes back.

That's an extra 2½ minutes on each end. It's not so much that you're going to be intimidated, but just enough to add duration to your run—and burn more fat and calories.

Start slower on your long run. Remember time is the goal, not distance.

If you have a running partner doing this program too, today

would be a good day to include both of you. Just make sure you run together, helping each other out, especially in that last extra minute of running.

Today is a day you do not want to run with people who are faster than you. The temptation will be to start too fast and end up walking before the halfway mark. Then you will be working backward, not forward.

So go ahead and run for 35 minutes.

Day Sixty-eight Log

Time: _____

Place: _____

Comments: _____

_____

_____

25 MINUTES

Today's Run

12 1/2 minutes out, 12 1/2 minutes back.

Create Your Own Log for the Future

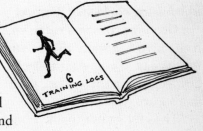

THIS BOOK is almost over, and you know what that means.

Time to create a running log of your own.

Your log will be a useful tool to further weight loss and help you keep running in several ways:

1 It gives you a record. And that helps you stay consistent, the key to this running/weight loss program.

2 It keeps you motivated. You can see the workouts you've done and the progress you've made. You'll want to keep running.

3 It tells you when to rest. Remember rest, a key tool in this running program? If you've gone more than a week without a rest day, you'll know it. And you can take a rest day and not feel guilty because of the workouts you see you've done before it on your log.

④ You can analyze what works and doesn't. If you feel like running hills again, you might want to look back in your log and see the last time you ran hills—and discover that the day after, your knee hurt. Maybe hills aren't for you.

⑤ It can help you look ahead. Write in goal workouts on your log weeks and months ahead of time. For instance, if you now are running 30 minutes without stopping, page ahead two months and write in 45 minutes, then see if you can get your workout up to that time.

To make your own running log you can use everything from pieces of scrap paper stapled together to computer disks to notebooks to daily planners to wall calendars—not to mention actual training log books like this one.

Choosing a medium for your log depends on you. All you really need is a space to write in the run each day and a number for the day. If you want to include more info (who ran with you, how you felt, what you had to eat afterward) pick something with more space.

The RUN AWAY FROM FAT book makes an excellent tool to do this. Just cross out the workout in the book and substitute your own new workout. And you can keep them on the shelf. So why not add to your collection?

Day Sixty-nine Log

Time: _____

Place: _____

Comments: _____

_____

_____

35 MINUTES

Today's Run

17 1/2 minutes out, 17 1/2 minutes back.

Testimonial

▪ ▪ ▪ ▪ ▪ ▪ ▪ ▪ ▪ ▪ ▪ ▪ ▪ ▪ ▪

MEET KRISTY. Maybe you know someone like her. This attractive 28-year-old sales rep likes to go out and have a good time on the weekends. Yet she continues to have less fat on her than a well-trimmed steak.

That's because, Kristy says, she has a secret weapon. "I run four or five times a week," she says. "I do that because I know running is the best way to burn calories and fat. But I also know the best way to get the most fat burning out of my running."

Let her explain. "I know that when I run, I can burn roughly 100 plus calories for every mile of running I do, and that's when I'm running pretty slow. I'll do a slow run for four or five miles a few times a week. But I also know that if I pick up the pace on some of my runs, I'll burn more fat, so twice a week I'll do pickups [see Day 72] during my runs where I increase the speed for 30 seconds to a minute, then slow down for a minute or two to rest, then pick up the speed again. I try for four or five of these.

"I find that these added speed runs are a great change of pace that also really help me stay trim.

"It's my secret to eating what I want and still looking the way I want to." (For more on pickups see Day 72.)

Day Seventy Log

Time: _____

Place: _____

Comments: _____

_____

_____

0 MINUTES

Today's Run

0 minutes.

Read About Running

▪ ▪ ▪ ▪ ▪ ▪ ▪ ▪ ▪ ▪ ▪ ▪ ▪ ▪ ▪ ▪

OKAY, YOU'VE been running for several weeks; your endurance is up; you're having a good time mixing workouts and running friends; and, most important, you've dropped a few pounds.

Hey, you say to yourself, this running thing is for me. Where do I learn more?

Well, in addition to this book, there are other publications that can teach you about running.

Runner's World magazine is the world's largest running magazine and the number-one authority on the sport. With more than half a million readers in the United States and another quarter million worldwide—in places like Great Britain, the Netherlands, Finland, Germany, South Africa, Australia, China—you know that *Runner's World* knows what it is talking about.

In *RW*'s pages you'll find everything from helpful hints on nutrition, health, motivation and, yes, weight loss to profiles of top runners and stories about major races all over the world. Its editors include a Boston Marathon champ and past Olympians. You can get it on the newsstand, by subscription or at your local library.

A second source is running books. There are too many to list here, but a short list includes the following:

Four Months to a Four-Hour Marathon, by Dave Kuehls. Perigee Books. 1998.

The Quotable Runner, edited by Mark Will-Weber. Breakaway Books. 1995.

The Runner's Book of Training Secrets, by Ken Sparks and Dave Kuehls. Rodale Press. 1996.

The Essential Runner, by John Hanc. Lyons & Bufford. 1995.

The Complete Book of Running, edited by Amby Burfoot. Rodale Press. 1997.

Day Seventy-one Log

Time: _____

Place: _____

Comments: _____
_____
_____

20 MINUTES/ PICKUPS

Today's Run

Jog for 7 minutes then run 3 times 60 seconds at a faster pace, jogging for one minute in between each (keep track of time on your sports watch). Jog 7 minutes to finish.

Fat-Burning Workout #3: Pickups

O KAY, YOU'VE been running steadily now for more than two months. What started as a 10-minute run has turned into a 35-minute run. You can see the weight loss you've accomplished already. You're going to keep gradually running more minutes to help melt the pounds away. You've run striders and a few hills and found out what a great fat burner those runs can be.

Are there any other ways you can increase fat burning?

There are. And one is called "pickups."

Pickups are gradual increases in speed spread out throughout your run. For instance, if you were going on a 30-minute run and you wanted to do 5 pickups during the run, you would first run an easy five minutes for a warmup. Then once every three minutes you would run a one-minute pickup.

By increasing your speed for just this little amount of time, you burn more calories than you would normally on an easy 30-minute run. Plus, you're cranking up your metabolism, and it takes time to come back down. So you benefit from what's known as the "after-burn effect"—burning more calories and fat after your run is over.

Plus, pickups lower your post-run appetite. So you not only burn more calories and fat; you are less hungry afterward, too.

The key to pickups is to find the right speed for you. The first time out, steadily increase your cadence by swinging your arms harder and pumping your knees, until you find yourself at a pace where you are breathing hard through your mouth. Now—using your stopwatch—try and stay at this pace for 60 seconds. If you have to slow down, maybe that pace is too fast. You should feel winded but not exhausted after the 60 seconds. Try for at least three 60-second pickups the first time out. Gradually build to 8 over a period of weeks.

Okay, now pick it up.

Day Seventy-two Log

Time: _____

Place: _____

Comments: _____

_____

_____

15 MINUTES

Today's Run

Out for 7 1/2 minutes, back for 7 1/2 minutes.

Blisters

PROBABLY THE most common problem for new runners, blisters can form on the back of the heel, bottom of the foot, between the toes, or anywhere there is friction when you run.

There are several causes for them and subsequent preventative measures:

1 Wearing new shoes that are not broken in. Always walk in new shoes before you go for a run in them. Never take them fresh out of the box and run for 25 minutes. You're inviting blisters.

2 New socks. As with shoes, socks have to be broken in. Don't put on a new pair of socks and then run for 30 minutes.

3 Dirty socks. Dirty socks don't absorb as much moisture as clean ones, and they start to bunch and rub your feet in certain areas, causing blisters.

4 Improperly fitting shoes. A shoe that rubs just a bit on the ankles when you try them on in a shoe store is a shoe that will cause a quarter-sized blister on your ankle by the end of a 30-minute run. Make sure there is plenty of room at the toes and that the ankles are not being rubbed. (A good preventative measure for blisters is to rub Vaseline between the toes and on the ankle before you run. This may feel gooey at first, but it does work.)

When you get a blister, you will feel a hot sensation in the area. There is not much you can do about it if it strikes you during your run. If it is too painful to continue running, just walk back.

After you go home take your shoes and socks off and examine the blister. A small blister—the size of a dime—might be best left alone. Just keep it clean, and it should go away soon.

If your blister is quarter-sized or more, you might want to lance it because it causes pain just walking on it. You can go to a clinic and get this done.

Or take care of the blister at home: Sterilize a needle with rubbing alcohol and slide the needle into the bottom of the blister—make sure you've washed the area thoroughly. Once you have punctured the blister, retract the needle and press on the top of the blister to draw all the fluid out. Dab with alcohol to sterilize and swab on some antibacterial ointment to prevent infection.

It's best not to run on a painful blister—running on it can just make it grow. But if you have to run, slather it with Vaseline to prevent more friction and wrap it in a gauze bandage. If you can get all that into your shoes and run without pain, go ahead.

Day Seventy-three Log

Time: _____

Place: _____

Comments: _____

_____

_____

30 MINUTES

Today's Run

Out for 15 minutes, back for 15 minutes.

The 150-Calorie Deficit

T HE GREAT thing about losing weight through running is that it's so easy to keep it off once you've lost it.

Because running to lose weight involves constant activity and calorie burning (unlike diets that just cut calories and then you're back to square one when you begin to eat again), you've actually got an insurance policy against gaining back that weight you've lost and the fat you've burned.

It's much more simple than you think.

You don't have to keep starving yourself—like many people when their 90-day diet ends. And you don't have to continually run more. All you have to do is eat sensibly and continue to run three to five days a week.

That's where the 150-calorie deficit comes in.

All that means is if you burn 150 calories more than you consume each day, you're in the golden zone, where you won't gain back any weight that day.

There are two ways to make sure you're always in the 150-calorie zone.

1 Keep running. This will keep your metabolism high and burn fat and calories daily.

2 Eat sensibly. Make wise food choices such as substituting mustard for mayonnaise or cut out a soda for lunch and substitute water and you've already cut out more than 150 calories for the day.

It's that simple. Just make sure you stay consistent in your running and eating habits, and don't binge on certain unhealthy foods, like pizza and ice cream, and you can keep the fat off indefinitely.

Day Seventy-four Log

Time: _____

Place: _____

Comments: _____

_____

_____

30 MINUTES

Today's Run

Out for 15 minutes, back for 15 minutes.

Injuries

■ ■ ■ ■ ■ ■ ■ ■ ■ ■ ■ ■ ■ ■ ■ ■

A GOOD code word to remember when dealing with any type of ankle or knee injury is RICE.

This is an abbreviation for helpful self-treatment.

For example, say on your run today you lost your footing and stepped in a small hole. You get back from your run and you feel your ankle starting to swell.

It's not too severe, but you want to be on the safe side without lugging yourself down to the clinic. You know the difference between a mild injury and a medical emergency.

So what do you do?

You RICE it.

R: First of all you need to REST. That means no running the next day, even if you've got a group run. You want the injury to heal not aggravate it.

I: The second thing is get some ICE on it as soon as possible. Ice helps bring down the swelling and aids in tissue repair. Try to ice the area for at least 10 minutes, no more than 15 minutes. Ice it four times a day. Use ice cubes in a plastic bag, or frozen peas, or a cold pack or ice cups (frozen water in a Dixie cup). The important thing is to ice it.

C: The next thing is COMPRESSION. If you are going to work the next day, make sure to wrap that ankle in an Ace bandage or ankle brace for extra support.

E: The last things you need to do and in many ways the most important if the ankle twist is more severe is ELEVATION. To reduce swelling 24 hours a day make sure your ankle is always up. Try to lie on a couch with your ankle propped up on pillows so it is above your heart. But if you can't do that, prop it up on anything handy. If you don't, the blood will pool and your ankle will swell and the damaged tissue does not get flushed out.

Day Seventy-five Log

Time: _____

Place: _____

Comments: _____

_____

_____

40 MINUTES

Today's Run

Out for 20 minutes, back for 20 minutes. You will be bumping up your time once again by 5 minutes. Makes sure you start out slow and that you run with a training partner to help motivate you.

New Shoes

TIME FOR a shoe check. Take a look at the pair you started with two and a half months ago.

They don't look as brightly colored do they? Perhaps there is some ground-in dirt or grass stains on them. Maybe the formerly white shoelaces look brown.

You know what? All that really doesn't matter. Most shoes will lose that new-shoe look in a matter of days or weeks.

What you really have to watch is the bottom of your shoes and, in a way, the inside of your shoes. That will tell you when it's time for new shoes.

Roughly, your shoes should last at least three to six months, maybe more, depending on what surface you run on (concrete will wear down shoes faster than grass). The easiest way to gauge wear and tear on your shoes is to look at the bottom, the soles.

Examine the treads. Are they all worn down? Do you in fact have smooth patches near the toes and heel?

If that is the case, then it's probably a pretty easy call to go get new shoes.

But what if the tread is not worn down? And you've been running for almost three months and you FEEL each time you put your foot down as if it's coming in direct contact with the ground—it feels as if there is no cushion left between your foot and the ground?

Then it's time to examine the midsole. When it comes to wear and tear the midsole is the most crucial part of the shoe.

The midsole is the foam or air or whatever is between the rubber sole and your foot. The midsole is what absorbs the shock of the impact of your foot hitting the ground several thousand times each run.

The midsole compresses like a mattress, then bounces back.

But over time that ability to bounce back decreases. And though you can't see anything wrong with your midsoles—there are no tears or hole—you'll feel as though you're running on dead legs.

There is no hard and fast test for midsole breakdown. You just have to trust your legs to tell you how they feel. If you've been following this program, after about six months you should be looking for a new pair of shoes.

It's time for new shoes after four months if you're running more than 30 minutes per day on average.

If you can afford it, always indulge yourself with new shoes. They are the best injury prevention money can buy. And they will also give more spring to your legs, so you can get out there and run away from fat!

Day Seventy-six Log

Time: _____

Place: _____

Comments: _____

_____

_____

30 MINUTES

Today's Run

Out for 15 minutes, back for 15 minutes.

Testimonial

· ■ ■ ■ ■ ■ ■ ■ ■ ■ ■ ■ ■

MEET DENISE. She's a 34-year-old mother.
Prior to her pregnancy she weighed a slim 120 pounds.
But after giving birth she stayed at 145 pounds. She wanted to do something about it.

"I tried walking at first, but that just seemed to take a lot of time, without the weight-loss results," she said.

Then she tried aerobics. "I could feel myself toning up but I still had a lot of weight to lose," she recalls.

Then one day she took a deep breath and went to the local running path half a mile from her health club. "I didn't know how far I was going, I just knew that I wanted to run," she recalls.

That first day Denise made it 10 minutes. But she kept at it—20 minutes, then 30 minutes, then 40 minutes—and the fat started disappearing.

After the weight came off, she felt—and looked—so good that she started wearing shorts and a jogging bra to run in. Denise was a 30-something mother and she was getting looks she hadn't gotten since her high school days.

Today, Denise is an avid runner: 4–5 days a week, 4–6 miles a day. "I'm hooked, but it's a healthy addiction," she says. "Running is by far the best way to lose weight and keep it off. If you are coming off a pregnancy, I highly recommend it."

Just be sure you check with your health care professional and are cleared for post-pregnancy exercise before you begin.

Day Seventy-seven Log

Time: _____

Place: _____

Comments: _____

_____

_____

0 MINUTES

Today's Run

0 minutes.

Walkmans

■   ■   ■   ■   ■   ■   ■   ■   ■   ■

NEW RUNNERS especially seem to want to use these as a crutch. You've seen other runners use them. They look like something a runner should use. Plus, if you have them on, you won't be embarrassed by having to talk to another runner when you are first starting out.

Well, all that makes no sense at all.

First of all, most of the runners you see using them are using them to make a fashion statement and nothing else.

Walkmans are not good for beginning runners because the negatives outweigh the pluses.

Pluses:

1 The only plus would be motivation from the music, but as you will see, there are other motivators better than music.

Negatives:

1 They add extra weight. You're trying to lose weight through running, and that is accomplished by running for more min-

utes, not by carrying around weights in your hands or strapped to your waistband.

2 They add extra hassle. Cords can get in the way. Stations can fade in and out. You end up stopping and starting and not really running for your 40 minutes.

3 They interfere with your learning how to run. If you are new to running, you are concentrating on proper running form, which includes how to hold your hands. You won't learn this if one hand is constantly clutching a radio.

4 It can be dangerous. You want all your senses alert when you are running. On streets you won't hear cars or pedestrians come up. On park trails you won't hear other runners or walkers or bicyclists. In both locales, you won't hear dogs.

5 They take away your awareness of your breathing and stride—the rhythm of the breath and feet that are so much a part of running.

6 They keep you from making new running friends. Nothing is harder to do on the run than to strike up a conversation with your Walkman on. You'll have to fiddle with the dials, and other runners will see your Walkman as an indication that you don't want to be bothered and pass on by without a word. You could miss meeting a training partner because of that.

7 Run time is clear thinking time. As you progress in your running program, you will find that you can do your clearest thinking while on the run. That's because oxygen is circulating to the brain. But if your brain is full of Mariah Carey's latest, what kind of thinking are you going to do?

Of course, if you absolutely, positively have to run with a Walkman—and, admittedly, there are many people who say this is so—go ahead. The bottom line is, if you wouldn't run without your Walkman, go ahead and use it. But if you can get by without it, get by without it. Just keep those negatives in mind, and maybe you can break yourself of the habit.

Day Seventy-eight Log

Time: _____

Place: _____

Comments: _____
_____
_____

20 MINUTES/ TEMPO RUN

Today's Run

Jog for 10 minutes, then run 3 minutes at tempo pace. Jog for 7 minutes.

Fat-Burning Trick #4: Tempo Runs

ANOTHER WAY to burn lots of fat during a run is to do a tempo run.

Tempo runs are great for everyone because they are geared to your tempo—and no one else's.

Roughly speaking, a tempo run would go like this: Warm up with a 10-minute slow jog, then shift into tempo pace. (This is roughly 85 percent effort, or a pace that makes you breathe a little harder but is not too uncomfortable. If you had to, you could hold tempo pace for pretty long.) Now run tempo pace for 3 minutes. Jog 7 minutes for a cooldown.

You've run for 20 minutes, but you've burned more fat and calories in those 20 minutes because you've upped the tempo for 3 minutes. You can gradually increase the time of your tempo run, say, by 2 minutes every 2 weeks until you're running 15 minutes tempo. This is a good limit because any more would make you too tired to run tomorrow.

Remember to increase the time of your tempo run, but don't

increase intensity (that is, don't try to run at your pickup pace). The entire tempo run should feel comfortably hard, not as if each step is your last. When you finish, you should feel exhilarated but not wiped out. But, if when you are running tempo pace, you find it suddenly hard to hold that pace, what do you do?

You slow down a little and keep running. The whole idea is to run for a faster pace for a certain amount of TIME. Constant effort, not speed, is the goal of this run.

Tempo runs, if done right, will make you stronger and burn tons of fat because the faster you run, the more total calories you burn—and that means burning more fat.

Following are some examples of different tempo runs you can run as your fitness level increases, eventually working up to a tempo run of 20 minutes (any more and you are taxing the body too much):

1. Jog for 10 minutes, then run 3 minutes at tempo pace. Jog for 7 minutes.

2. Jog for 5 minutes, then run 5 minutes at tempo pace. Jog for 5 minutes.

3. Jog for 5 minutes, then run 10 minutes at tempo pace. Jog for 5 minutes.

4. Jog for 5 minutes then run 15 minutes at tempo pace. Jog for 5 minutes.

5. Jog for 5 minutes then run 20 minutes at tempo pace. Jog for 5 minutes.

Tempo runs are also perfect when you are pressed for time. If you only have 15 minutes to run and your normal run on that day would be 30 minutes, you can do a 10-minute tempo run (warming up first with a 5-minute jog), and you'll burn just as much fat as you would on that 30-minute run.

That said, why don't we do tempo runs every day?

The answer is simple: They are a mildly stressful run and you need two or three easy days to recover from them, or else you'll find yourself injured or too tired to run.

Then what will you do? Sit at home and eat.

So go out today and do the first tempo run from the list above.

Day Seventy-nine Log

Time: _____

Place: _____

Comments: _____

_____

_____

25 MINUTES

Today's Run

Out for 12 1/2 minutes, back for 12 1/2 minutes.

Making Time to Run

I F YOU are like most people, every day is a busy day.

I've already told you that the ideal time to run is after work, when you're winding down from the day and preparing for a nice evening.

But that doesn't always work out.

There are other ways to fit a run into your schedule.

Morning

Most of us work 9–5, so mornings might be time for an occasional run. You accomplish this in five ways.

1 Go to bed earlier the night before: half an hour or an hour earlier. Wind down with a cup of hot milk. Get into bed and relax. You're trying to change your sleeping patterns here, so take it easy.

2 Wake up with everything ready to go: Mornings are going to be rush time. So when that alarm clock goes off at 5:30 a.m., you should have your shoes and shorts and socks and singlet (or T-shirt) already laid out on a chair before you.

Splash some water on your face, go to the bathroom, drink a glass of water, head out the door.

3 Meet a friend: Morning runs are easier if you have arranged to meet with a running partner. That will give you motivation to get out of bed and out the door.

4 Have work clothes ready when you get back. Shower and dress.

5 Have breakfast already out: a bowl of cereal, banana and a glass of juice . . . and you're out the door.

Lunchtime or During the Day

Lunch hour is a good time to get in a run if you have adequate changing and shower facilities at work or a gym nearby. During the day—for college students and mothers at home—is also a good time to run (though mothers at home might want to bargain with their husbands so that he watches the kids in the evening while she runs).

The trick is, like in the morning, having everything ready. That means bringing running clothes to work, going straight to the gym at lunch to change, then out to the track or trail. Then it's back to the gym to shower and still have time to grab a healthy sandwich at the deli.

Late Nights

Not recommended, except as a last-ditch effort. Anytime you run past 8 p.m., you are going to interfere with getting to sleep that night because running energizes you. You'll feel calm and tired, but you will have a tougher time getting to sleep if you've run late at night.

Plus, it can be dangerous outside after dark. So if you have to run late at night, make sure to run with friends and wear a reflective vest or clothing, or run in a health club.

Day Eighty Log

Time: _____

Place: _____

Comments: _____

_____

_____

30 MINUTES

Today's Run

15 minutes out, 15 minutes back.

Black Toenails

▪ ▪ ▪ ▪ ▪ ▪ ▪ ▪ ▪ ▪ ▪ ▪ ▪ ▪ ▪ ▪

A COMMON malady for beginning runners is black toe-nails.

Generally this problem happens to the toenail on either big toe, but it can happen to any toe-nail.

What happens is that a blood blister forms beneath the nail, causing the nail to become black because of the blood underneath.

Black toenails, while not serious, can be plenty painful at the initial stages because of the pressure exerted on the nail from the blood blister. If the pressure is too intense, you can go to a clinic where a doctor will release the pressure for you.

A home remedy is to take a sterilized needle and puncture the nail, releasing the blood and fluid.

If all this sounds icky to you, it is. And a much better way of dealing with black toenails is to prevent them.

Black toenails are caused by not having enough room in the toe box of your shoes or running too much downhill—forcing your toes to hit the front of your shoes repeatedly.

To prevent this from happening, when you buy your shoes make sure there is 1/2 inch between your toes and the front of the shoe. This will give your toes room to move on the run.

Also, limit downhill running if you feel pressure being exerted on your toes.

Remember also to clip your nails regularly. This will keep them from hitting the front of your shoes.

If you do all these things, you shouldn't have a run-in with black toenails.

Day Eighty-one Log

Time: _____

Place: _____

Comments: _____

_____

_____

40 MINUTES

Today's Run

Out for 20 minutes, back for 20 minutes.

Mental Running

■   ■   ■   ■   ■   ■   ■   ■   ■   ■   ■   ■   ■

SURE, RUNNING and weight loss are mostly physical. Just ask your tired legs and body after a good 35-minute run.

But what many experienced runners learn is that once you get going with a running program, it's 90 percent mental.

What does that mean?

That means the success of your running routine—and weight-loss goals—will depend on how you approach each day's run mentally. There will be physical cues, such as feeling the need to run. On some days when you can't run, you will find, surprisingly, that you miss it. And if you've grown accustomed to running at a certain time during the day, say, right after work, your body will be secretly preparing for your run.

But all that will not help as much as being mentally prepared for your run.

Mental running starts long before you hit the trail or road or treadmill. Say, for instance, that you are going to run 40 minutes after work on a nearby trail. This 40-minute run will be the farthest you have run yet. So when the alarm rings in the morning, you've already got this goal in mind for you today.

Take a look at the training log part of this book. See how far you have progressed in the past months. This will pump you up and get you subconsciously focused during the day on your run.

At your coffee break, talk to a few friends about your upcoming run. Stating a goal, psychologists tell us, is a good step toward achieving it.

At lunch, buy a high-carbohydrate snack to set aside for later in the afternoon—it will provide the energy burst that's going to carry you through your run.

In the afternoon take time out and see yourself running on the trail, running farther and farther than you have run before. Smell the trees and feel the wind in your face. This is called imaging. And you can use it daily.

Finally, right before you start your run, touch some physical cue, like a tree or a bench. Then tell yourself you are going to run out for 20 minutes, turn around, and come back to this very spot—to touch it.

This, in effect, grounds your goal to something physical, convincing you that your run is not just a part of you, but a part of the world around you.

And that's mental running.

Day Eighty-two Log

Time: _____

Place: _____

Comments: _____

_____

_____

40 MINUTES

Today's Run

20 minutes out, 20 minutes back.

When You Don't Feel Like Running

■ ■ ■ ■ ■ ■ ■ ■ ■ ■ ■ ■ ■ ■ ■

N O MATTER how gradually you build up your running program by following the specific workouts in this book, no matter how mentally prepared you get for each day's run, some days you will just not feel like running. It won't be because of physical pain. (If you are suffering physically, you should not be running. And it won't be fatigue. If you are overly fatigued, you should take a day off.)

Maybe you are starting to "feel" a little burned out on the "routine."

What should you do?

There are several possibilities:

1 Plan a group run that meets once or twice a week. Really make it an event, with dinner out afterward.

2 Run in a park you have never run before.

3 If you don't normally, take your dog along.

4 Enter a Fun Run. Look for local road races in the newspaper or check with your local running group. Most 10Ks have

a Fun Run of a mile or two before the main event. Go there and register. Run the race, and if you feel like running more, get an extra five or 10 minutes. (This is a great way to meet new training partners.) Also, if you have a race planned for the future—say three weeks ahead—this will help you continue your running program.

5 Buy yourself a cheap trophy and have it waiting for you at the end of your run. You could even have it engraved: "First Place Tuesday Night Run." Or "You Made It—You've Lost Seven Pounds—Now Let's Eat a Healthy Meal," something like that.

The trick is to anticipate the malaise. After a week or a few days you may feel yourself starting to grind. You won't look forward to your runs like you did last month (even the mental prep tips aren't getting you over the edge). You're not burned out yet, but you can feel it coming.

THAT'S when you get on the horn to some friends and plan a group run two days from now.

And that's how you head burnout off at the pass.

And that's how you keep running away from fat.

Day Eighty-three Log

Time: _____

Place: _____

Comments: _____

_____

_____

30 MINUTES

Today's Run

Out for 15 minutes, back for 15 minutes.

Testimonial

■ ■ ■ ■ ■ ■ ■ ■ ■ ■ ■ ■ ■ ■ ■

M EET KATHY. After two kids she still has the body of a 19-year-old. This 35-year-old mother crams a lot into every day, and a run is one of them.

"It's what I look forward to in the afternoon when my husband comes home," she says. "I say, 'Your turn to watch the kids.' Just give me 45 minutes to an hour and I can change, run, shower and change back. That's all I need."

Of course, when Kathy had just one child, she often took the baby on runs with her in the baby jogger. "It's really not as complicated or tough as it looks; it almost pulls you along at times."

And once a week, Mom watches the kids so Kathy can accompany her husband on a five-mile run, after which they go out for a healthy dinner. "It's the Wednesday night special: no kids, a nice run with my husband and a nice relaxing meal afterward. What could be better?"

And running, Kathy found, was the best way to lose the weight she had gained from her pregnancy. "It was the most time-effective fat and calories burner I've found. I was a competitive swimmer for years, and I never thought I'd be hooked on another exercise, but I am. Running is for me."

Day Eighty-four Log

Time: _____

Place: _____

Comments: _____

_____

_____

0 MINUTES

Today's Run

0 minutes.

Enter a 5K

■ ■ ■ ■ ■ ■ ■ ■ ■ ■ ■ ■ ■ ■ ■ ■

CONGRATULATIONS. YOU'RE just about finished with this program. 90 days. That's more than 12 weeks. Three months. Now comes the big question. What do I do next?

If you've been keeping up with this program, you'll want to continue to expand your running horizons because running has helped you lose weight. It has also made you feel good and given you more energy. In short, you want to continue running because running is now a part of your life.

So what's the next step?

You can gradually build up your timed runs or increase the intensity of the ones you run now or seek out new places to run and people to run with. Or you can continue your comfortable routine. Or you can race.

Before you get so nervous about the idea of racing that you drop this book, let's look at racing as an option.

To keep running fresh and interesting, many runners do races every so often. The shortest distance—a 5K, 3.1 miles—is short enough that you've probably already covered it in practice, so why not try it in a race? The only difference is that you won't be running alone or with a friend but, maybe, with thousands of other runners.

To find a 5K, check out the local paper from the spring to the fall or visit a running shoe store or contact the local running club.

There should be plenty of races. Find one nearby and on a day when you don't have a thousand things planned. You can send away for an application or preregister through the mail, saving a few bucks. (Most races cost between $8 and $12.) Or register the morning of the race for a few dollars more.

If you do register the morning of the race, make sure to arrive an hour before race time to give yourself enough time to register and then get warmed up for the race. Most races will also give you a race T-shirt and other knickknacks. You can also pick up applications for future races.

Okay, here's what you need to know for your first race. Make sure to line up in the back of the pack. The faster runners move to the front, and if you start with them, two things can happen and they are both bad: 1) You sprint out with the fast guys and end up walking half a mile into the race. 2) You start slow and get trampled by the faster runners behind you.

The most important thing about racing your first 5K—and all races for that matter—is: Don't start running too fast. You'll be keyed up with adrenaline, so force yourself to run slow at the starting gun. Try to maintain a comfortable pace for at least 2 miles. Then, if you still feel like running faster, you can pick up the pace. That way, you won't end up walking in your first race. You'll finish strong, crossing the line proud.

So spend today looking for information on a race to run next month.

Day Eighty-five Log

Time: _____

Place: _____

Comments: _____

_____

_____

15 MINUTES

Today's Run

Run out for 7 1/2 minutes, then back for 7 1/2 minutes. Do this run in the evening after a light dinner. Drink lots of water, but do not eat again before bedtime. Get up in the morning and do the second half of the workout on Day 87.

Fat-Burning Workout #5: PM/AM

A N ADVANCED running workout to Run Away From Fat is the PM/AM.

Here's the workout.

The evening before your morning run eat an early, light dinner and 2 hours later go for an easy 15-minute run. Then come home and drink lots of water, but go to bed without eating again.

The next morning—before breakfast—go out and run for 40 minutes straight or run hills, pickups or a tempo run. You can choose any one of your special Fat-Burning Workouts.

The strategy behind this dual workout is simple. The evening workout gets your metabolism burning through the night, and in the morning your body will be low on carbohydrates (your body's preferred fuel during runs), so the morning run will force your body to burn fat sooner in your workout and burn more fat than it normally would.

In that sense the AM/PM run is almost like squeezing fat out of your body. Just make sure to drink plenty of fluids in the morning and realize that your morning run will seem twice as hard because you're running on empty.

Then fuel back up with a hearty, carbohydrate-rich breakfast.

Day Eighty-six Log

Time: _____

Place: _____

Comments: _____
_____
_____

day eighty-seven

CHOOSE

Today's Run Second Half AM/PM

Run your favorite fat-burning workout. Choose among striders, hills, pickups and tempo runs.

Where Do I Go from Here?

■ ■ ■ ■ ■ ■ ■ ■ ■ ■ ■ ■ ■ ■

YOUR 90-DAY Run Away From Fat Program is just about over. You've lost weight, gained fitness and confidence. You started out struggling to run for 10 minutes, and now you can make 40 minutes at a time.

But where do you go from here?

It depends on what your ultimate goals are. You have several options:

1 40 minutes is the goal we worked up to for good reason. It is a great "mean" for fat burning and calorie consuming. You could keep your daily average at 40 minutes and continue to lose weight for the next 90 Days . . . and the next 90 Days.

You can't go wrong when you run 40 minutes at a time 5 or 6 days a week. You will lose more weight as long as you watch what you eat.

2 You can start another 90-Day Program that gradually ratchets up your time. A good "doable" goal would be to reach the point where you can run for an hour without stopping at the end of the next 90-Day segment. An hour is another good time goal because it burns major fat and so once you reach that,

you can make your hour run a special run—once a week—to burn fat and calories. And then devote the other 5 running days to shorter workouts. (Maybe start entering a race or two each month for fun. See "A Day at the Races," Day 89.)

Just remember to increase your running time in small doses. For example, for the first 45 days you can work up to getting comfortably running for 50 minutes and then for the next 45 days work up to your hour run. Remember to go slow on these runs because you are working to increase your "time spent running" and up your endurance so that your shorter runs will feel easier, and your intense runs that you do once a week—hills, pickups, tempo runs, and so on—will feel smoother and smoother.

The key is to work out a program that fits into your schedule and one that you like doing. That is the way you will keep Running Away From Fat.

3 There is a third option, although it's one I can't recommend: You can quit running. Satisfied with losing 5, 10, 15 pounds or more over the last 90 days?

Hey! You did it. Time to take a break, right? Grab a pizza and some ice cream to celebrate.

And watch those pounds come back faster than a boomerang.

The choice is yours, but since you've become a runner, why not stay one?

Day Eighty-seven Log

Time: _____

Place: _____

Comments: _____

_____

_____

CROSS-TRAIN/ 20 MINUTES

Today's Run

Cross-train for 20 minutes.

Cross That Line: Cross-Training

OKAY, I know. You're tired from yesterday's run. It's raining cats and dogs outside. And there's a line three deep at the health club treadmills. You want to run 20 minutes today, are scheduled to run that far, but in 30 minutes you have to be showered and changed and at the restaurant. What do you do?

This is a good time to talk about the benefits of cross-training.

Cross-training means substituting a like exercise for your run that day. It could be cycling or the StairMaster (the two best). Or it could be aerobics class or maybe some fast walking.

The point is, cross-training can be a valuable tool to keeping your Run Away From Fat Program going. Just make sure you don't stray away from your running too much. A good rule is to use cross-training when the weather is too bad to run or when you can't get out until dark or when you need a little break—say, once every two weeks.

Because, as I've stated earlier, running is the best, most efficient way to burn calories and fat and lose weight. But the only way you can do that is to keep running for weeks and months, and that's where cross-training can help.

Let's look at some of the cross-training options:

1. Cycling: A great cross-training alternative because it gets you sitting down, taking a little break from the constant up-rightness of running. It's a good break for your hips, knees and ankles because cycling is not a weight-bearing exercise. Cycle for 10 minutes longer than your scheduled run that day for a good cross-training workout. You might want to wear special bike shorts with extra padding to avoid "saddle sores."

2. StairMaster: Go five minutes longer on the StairMaster than you would for your run that day. Make sure you don't grasp the bars beside you, but swing your arms as if you were running uphill.

3. Aerobics: Try for a whole class period. They are generally 45 minutes.

4. Swimming: Half an hour of swimming, if you're not used to it, will be a great workout for your arms and lungs. Just keep out of the fast lanes so you don't get swum over.

Day Eighty-eight Log

Time: _____

Place: _____

Comments: _____

_____

_____

25 MINUTES

Today's Run

12 1/2 minutes out, 12 1/2 minutes back.

A Day At the Races

IF YOU are interested in jumping in some races with your new-found fitness, here is a rundown on the most popular distances and events:

Fun Runs

Held in conjunction with the main road race, such as a 5K or 10K, fun runs are "people runs" in the best sense of the word. Many entrants walk, most jog, a few run fast, but there is no real competition because awards aren't handed out. Everyone completes the distance "for fun."

Distances range from half a mile to 2 miles.

5K

The most popular race distance in the world. And for good reason. A 5K is 3.1 miles long, a distance that the beginning runner can complete. A 5K should take anywhere between 30 and 45 minutes for a new runner who is running to lose weight.

5 Miles

A popular road race distance also. Look to run between 45 and 60 minutes for a 5-mile run. This distance is doable if you have worked up to 50 minutes in practice.

10K

Twice a 5K, that is, 6.2 miles. Look to finish in an hour to 75 minutes. This distance is doable if you have worked up to an hour in practice.

15K

9.3 miles. A rare road race, but if you enter, look to finish in 90 minutes or more. You should not attempt this distance unless you have run for 80 minutes in practice.

Half-Marathon

13.1 miles. Look to finish in over two hours. A good goal for the beginning runner. Do not attempt to run this unless you've gone at least 10 miles in practice.

The Marathon

Oprah did it. She worked up to it for a long while, but she did it. For most people, a marathon will take at least 4 hours. Do not attempt this race unless you've gone through a marathon training program, like the ones outlined in my book, *4 Months to a 4-Hour Marathon*.

Day Eighty-nine Log

Time: _____

Place: _____

Comments: _____

_____

_____

40 MINUTES

Today's Run

20 minutes out, 20 minutes back.

Congratulations

■ ■ ■ ■ ■ ■ ■ ■ ■ ■ ■ ■ ■

YOU DID it. You Ran Away From Fat for 90 Days. You've probably lost a lot of weight, plus you've established a healthy lifestyle for the rest of your life.

Throughout this book you've read stories of people who have used running to lose weight. Guess what?

Now it's your turn.

This space is reserved for YOUR TESTIMONIAL.

_____

_____

_____

_____

_____

_____

_____

_____

_____

_____

_____

INDEX